T0171402

Hippocrates Is Not Dead

An Anthology of Hippocratic Readings

Patrick Guinan M.D.

University of Illinois-Chicago
College of Medicine

authorHOUSE®

AuthorHouse™
1663 Liberty Drive
Bloomington, IN 47403
www.authorhouse.com
Phone: 1-800-839-8640

First published by AuthorHouse   5/23/2011

ISBN: 978-1-4567-3544-9 (e)
ISBN: 978-1-4567-3545-6 (hc)
ISBN: 978-1-4567-3546-3 (sc)

Library of Congress Control Number: 2011903014

Printed in the United States of America

DEDICATION

1.) SEDES SAPIENTIA
The Source of Wisdom

2.) DR. HERBERT RATNER
Emphasizing the Wisdom of Nature in Medicine

3.) MY PARENTS
For Their Respect For, and Love of, Wisdom

Patrick Guinan is a Clinical Associate Professor in the Department of Urology of University of Illinois College of Medicine. He is the President of the Catholic Physicians Guild of Chicago. He graduated from the Medical College of Wisconsin and lives in Chicago.

TABLE OF CONTENTS

CONTRIBUTORS	CREDITS
Patrick Guinan, MD Clinical Associate Professor of Urology, University of Illinois College of Medicine	**Preface**
Leon Kass, MD Addie Clark Harding Professor, University of Chicago	**"Treatment Paragraphs"** "Is There a Medical Ethic"? In Toward a More Natural Science. Free Press, New York City, NY 1985, pp 224-246
Herbert Ratner, MD Co Founder National Commission On Human Life	**"Hippocrates Has Vital Meaning for Physicians"** General Practitioner, August, 1953, pp 93-99
John F. Brehany, PhD Executive Director Catholic Medical Association	**"The Indispensability of Hippocrates"** Presented at the CMA Region VII Symposium Mundelein, IL May 12, 2007.
Edmund Pellegrino, MD Former Chairman, Presidents Council On Bioethics	**"A Philosophical Basis for the Patient-Physician Interaction"** In: Toward a Reconstruction of Medical Morality, J of Med and Phil, 4:32-56, 1979.

INTRODUCTION

This book is about medicine, or more specifically, about the tradition of Medicine as expressed in the 2500 years of the Hippocratic ethic.

It is directed principally to those attracted to and beginning medical training (pre-med and medical students). But it will hopefully have appeal to practicing physicians, those caught up in administrative medicine and even the general public.

The philosophy of medicine is addressed specifically by Drs. Kass, Pellegrino and Cameron. This has to do with the covenantal relationship between a physician and patient. Drs. Ratner, Riley and Guinan emphasized the need for physicians to recognize the importance of working with nature and not becoming overly enamored with technology and pharmacology. Finally Dr. Brehany and Mr. Beeman discussed the more practical aspects of the ethics of medicine in a culturally materialistic society.

HIPPOCRATES BOOK

Preface

Why a book on Hippocrates? Isn't Hippocrates "dead"? Medical ethics, as exemplified by the 2500 year Hippocratic ethic and medical tradition, no longer guides the medical aspects of our culture. Its influence even on physicians and medical education is slowly being eroded.

While the Hippocratic ethic has guided medicine for 2500 years, since the 1970's bioethics, as a separate discipline, has dominated most areas of health care. The date of the eclipse of medical ethics by bioethics can rather clearly be set at April 18, 1979 when the Belmont Report was issued.[1]

Bioethics fulfilled the social need for a theory to resolve rising moral issues in the health care areas. These areas included health care financing, trans-plantation, human research protections, and dialysis, among many others. The Hippocratic ethic was felt to be too deontologic. That is, its guidelines were too strict and precluded what were, to be blunt, desired under the new cultural emphasis on the principle of autonomy. Paternalistic

---

1   The Belmont Report: Ethical Principles and Guidelines for the protection of Human Subjects for Research.
(Washington, D.C., Government Printing Office, 1979.

medicine was too autocratic. Bioethics was a perfect fit for the consensus democracy in the United States.

Opinion polls trumped Hippocratic principles. In the Belmont Report, the United States Congress had a compromise that applied consequentialist ethics to medical moral questions. This, it was argued, was the only approach available in a pluralistic society.

Bioethics may be a viable solution for broadly societal issues such as the care of the disabled and elderly and the financing of overall health care delivery.

But medicine is not, in its essence, societal. It is individual. The hallmark of the Hippocratic tradition is the doctor-patient relationship. That term may have a pejorative connotation today. But given its 2500 year staying power there is something basically human in the contract or healing covenant between a competent physician and a suffering patient. The Congressional Act approving the Belmont Report, which in essence inaugurated the new field of "bioethics". will not replace the Hippocratic doctor-patient relationship and traditional medical ethics.

In point of fact, suffering human persons have always and, in particular, need now, a personal one-on-one healing relationship with a competent physician. Bioethics cannot, and will not substitute for it.

Bioethics not only determines health care policies, but it, and not traditional Hippocratic medical ethics, is being taught in the United Sates Medical Schools. Beauchamp and Childress' "Principles of Biomedical Ethics"[2] is the most widely used ethic book by medical students.[3]

In an effort to refresh and promote the Hippocratic tradition we have published a series of essays dealing with Hippocrates and the Hippocratic ethic. It is intended principally for medical students but also for anyone else interested in the area of the ethics of medicine.

---

2   Beauchamp, Thomas and Childress, James. Principles of Biomedical Ethics, 5th Ed. (Oxford: Oxford University Press, 2001).
3   Du Bois, J.M. and Burkemper J. "Ethics Education in United States Medical Schools: a Study of Syllabi," Academic Medicine: 77 (May 2002), pp 432-447.

CHAPTER 1

TREATMENT PARAGRAPHS

By

Leon Kass, MD

The Content of the Oath: The Treatment Paragraphs. Let us begin, not illogically, with the passage that states the physician's main business: "I will apply dietetic measures for the benefit of the sick according to my ability and judgment; I will keep them from harm and injustice." This states unequivocally that it is sick individuals, not society or mankind or some abstract idea, who are the beneficiaries of the physician's activity. Moreover, the sick qualify for his services because they are sick, not because they have claims, desires, wishes, demands, or rights. The healer works with and for those who need to be healed, those who are not whole.

"Dietetic measures," once the main staple of the physician's therapeutic offerings, now strikes us as anachronistic, what with our cornucopia of pharmaceuticals, machines, and surgical procedures. Still, there are numerous medical conditions--including diabetes, hypertension, ulcers, heart failure, and gout--in which a dietary regimen is a central part of therapy and many others in which we suspect that diet is important, both as a cause of illness and as a cure.

Symptoms of malnutrition and starvation, as well as infections that feed on the malnourished are prevalent over much of the globe; symptoms and diseases caused or exacerbated by obesity are common in the prosperous countries. And if we broaden "dietetic" to mean "ingestibles," so as to include alcohol and other toxic substances as well as contaminated or despoiled foods, we see that regulation of diet still plays and will everywhere play a decisive role in benefiting the sick. We are, in a sense, what we eat.

But the Oath's emphasis on dietetic measures bespeaks a deeper teaching about the nature of medicine. What, after all, is diet or nutrition? It is the steady provision of necessary materials steadily consumed for energy or transformed from other to same by the body in metabolism, by which the body maintains in organized equilibrium its own functioning integrity. The ancients, in their naiveté, spoke of a balance of the four elements or humors; Claude Bernard, in his sophistication, taught us of homeostasis of the *milieu interieur*, the internal environment. Each implied that the healthy state is a certain balance or harmony of parts or elements that— and this is the crucial point – *the healthy harmonized body will produce on its own,* provided it acquires the right materials and is not obstructed, say, by superior invasive forces. *The body is its own healer,* and the physician a cooperative but subordinate partner who supplies the needed materials- whether it be protein or insulin, vitamin C or interferon, and by extension, even antibiotics to help the body arrest invasive obstruction from without. I do not insist that all current treatments can be rationalized on this homely model of supplying the necessaries, nor do I mean to assert that health is homeostasis-though I do think the time is ripe for a return to these philosophical matters. Rather, I mean to emphasize the Hippocratic Oath's tacit assertion that medicine is a cooperative rather than a transforming art, and that the physician is but an assistant to nature working within, the body having its own powerful (even if not invincible) tendencies toward healing itself (e.g., wound healing and other regenerative activities, or the rejection of foreign bodies and the immune response). Though our current technical prowess tends to make us forget these matters, does not the Oath speak truly?

The inherent tendencies toward wholeness are much more precarious in human beings than in our animal friends and relations. Our dietary habits are not given by instinct but by convention, habit, and choice. Man is the animal most likely to make himself sick, in the very act whose purpose is to nourish and sustain.

Sometimes we eat ourselves sick through ignorance of what is good for us, sometimes through incontinence and lack of self-restraint in the face of knowing better. In both these ways, we do ourselves unwitting harm and even injustice; that is, we treat ourselves unfittingly and worse than we deserve. The physician, according to the Oath, is not only one who brings a corrective diet to the already sick. He is also the one who seeks to prevent the ignorant and the self-indulgent from harming themselves. He has the knowledge needed to direct and inform the otherwise dangerously open and uninformed human appetites. It may at first seem strange to think that we human beings need such knowledgeable outsiders or that we do not know what is good for us, all the more so on the premise that our body is the primary healer and the doctor but the physician's assistant. But a body possessed of the power of reason, and hence also of choice, is a body whose possessor may lead it astray, owing to ignorance or wayward impulse. The physician, the ally of our body and of those inner powers working toward our own good, supplies needed knowledge, advice, and exhortation. He seeks to keep us from self-harm and injustice. The Oath's little paragraph on dietetics, properly unpacked, reveals the core of medicine.

The mention of the injustice that a person can do to himself becomes the link to the next provision, the one that forswears giving deadly drugs or abortifacients. This provision, I have already suggested, wisely implies that the true physician will not use his available means indiscriminately, to promote alien ends. The physician is no mere technician, selling his services on demand. But what is a proper and what an alien end? If the goal is to benefit the sick, what are the limits of "benefit"? The present passage shows us how to think about this, for the limits on the use of technique are derived from an understanding of the essence of the healing activity.

The forswearing of both giving a deadly drug if asked and making such a suggestion shows that the provision has suicide and active euthanasia in mind, rather than, say, a self-imposed restraint on murder or poisonings. The doctor refuses to participate directly in ending a life, whether one in the fullness of days or on the way to birth. To protect life, to maintain and support it, to restore it to wholeness, and certainly not to destroy it, is the common principle. To be sure, this principle gets outside support from religious teachings, pagan and Judeo-Christian. But, in our context, one sees that it can be derived from the inner meaning of medicine itself, especially if one remembers that the doctor is nature's cooperative ally and not its master. Is it not self-contradictory for the healing art to be the killing art--even in those cases in which we might all agree that killing is not murder (i.e., that it is legitimate)? Consider, for example, recent statutes in several states that, for reasons of humanity and economy, make injection of poison, rather than electrocution, the method of capital punishment. Put aside, for the moment, your reservations about capital punishment itself, and consider only whether physicians, if asked, ought to agree to administer the injections? Would that action be compatible with the medical vocation? I should say not. (Interestingly, at least for now, both the statutes and the medical profession agree with this conclusion. The statutes say that the injection shall not be made by a physician, and the AMA, I understand, has voted its official opposition to physician participation in such activities.)

Abortions are now performed by many doctors. I am aware that their uniform refusal to do so, were that to occur, would in practice nullify the "freedom to abort" that flowed from the Supreme Court's 1973 decision in Roe v. Wade (though, in fact, the overturning of legislative prohibitions on abortions did not oblige doctors to perform them). But the question before us here is not the morality or legality of abortion, but whether physicians who perform them are truly physicians. Set aside your opinions about abortion as such, and consider only whether the destruction of nascent life – life to which obstetricians give prenatal care, and whose needs are increasingly studied with a view to improving such care – is compatible with the inner meaning of medicine. If medicine is a technique neutral regarding the end, then the act of womb-emptying performed by obstetrical technique is equally properly used for birth and feticide. But if medicine is constituted by the task to assist living nature in human bodies to the work of maintenance and function and perpetuation, then one must wince at the monstrous self-contradictory union that is the obstetrician- abortionist. (I shall refrain from considering whether proper medical ministering to female humanity is finally compatible with assisting women in abortion, for reasons having to do not with fetal life but with the meaning of womanhood. The question, admittedly complex, is whether in opting for abortion a woman is doing harm or injustice to herself as a woman [i.e., by contradicting her generative nature] however much it may serve her wishes or aspirations as a [gender- free] human being.)

Perhaps I am mistaken in deriving these restraints strictly from the meaning of medicine. The end of this paragraph reads: "In purity and holiness I will guard my life and my art." What have purity and especially holiness to do with medicine?

Moreover, the syntax might suggest that they are invoked as extrinsic principles, *outside* of "my life and my art," to guide how one lives one's life and how one uses one's art. It is especially this statement that led Ludwig Edelstein to conclude that the Oath is a Pythagorean and not simply a physician's oath, or, in other words, that the ethical teachings of the Oath are brought *to* medicine from some universalist (though sectarian) teaching rather than derived *from* the particular (though universal) nature of healing itself. I shall return to this question later.

The last of the three paragraphs on treatment forswears surgery, even in the face of the most excruciating pain. But it does so not, as in the previous case, because the relief of such suffering violates the meaning of medicine, but because the physician does not specialize in surgery. One might wonder whether the physicians of the Oath drew back from the knife because they regarded surgery as a mutilation or at least a violation of bodily wholeness, incompatible with their ministerial function. Surgery, however much it shares the goals of the medicine of diet and drug, is in its nature aggressive, invasive, and assaulting. Even today, we note differences between surgeons and internists in their stance and attitude toward the body. Nevertheless, it is unlikely that the Hippocratic physician forswears surgery as a violation of the medical spirit or, for that matter, of purity or holiness.

For if this were his reason, he would not endorse the practice of surgery by those who do it. The physician is, rather, promising not to try himself to do what he cannot do, even in the face of a most severe suffering that might tempt his intervention. He willingly turns those in need over to someone competent in the necessary extra medical skill; the Oath thereby also teaches that we do not simply abandon those we cannot help ourselves. Cynical people may see here the beginning of specialization, trade restriction, fee-splitting, and the like, but the context favors a higher interpretation: Know your limits and let not your wishes to help exceed your competence to do so. Good intentions are dangerous if not coupled to competence. Who could disagree?

Today, it is true, surgery has been brought fully into the medical domain--though in Britain surgeons are still referred to as "mister" while other physicians are called "doctor," and a leading American medical school still distinguishes them in calling itself the College of Physicians and Surgeons. The knife for the stone is now a part of medicine. But today there are other areas and concerns pressing in on physicians, asking them to lend a hand. People oppressed in spirit or transgressing the law, people who beat their children or are beaten in love, people who fail in school or in life all ask the doctor to wield a new kind of knife he either does not have or cannot use with reasonable hope of success. With the proper updating, for swearing the knife still makes sense. It is only partly an excuse to say that there are no others who "are engaged in this work." Acting incompetently from good intentions is often worse than doing nothing, especially in the increasing number of instances in which the offer of pills and other forms of medical assistance for what are fundamentally problems of living fosters the false and enfeebling expectation that life itself has a technical solution.

CHAPTER 2

HIPPOCRATES HAS VITAL MEANING FOR PHYSICIANS

By

Herbert Ratner, MD

"WHY is it that doctors, although they admire Hippocrates, do not read his writings, or if by chance they do, do not understand them, or if they have the good fortune to understand them, do not put their principles into practice and develop the habit of their use?" It was six centuries after Hippocrates that the great Galen asked this of his contemporaries in an address entitled "That the Good Physician Is a Philosopher."

The timelessness of Galen's observation is in part communicated by his reference to a perennial sports event: "The fate reserved for the majority of athletes who, while aspiring to win victory in the Olympic games, do nothing in order to attain it, applies equally well to the majority of doctors. These last, indeed, praise Hippocrates, regarding him as first in the art of healing, yet they do everything except what should be done to resemble him."

The timelessness is better substantiated by the high role Hippocrates has played through the ages. It is of note that when William Harvey, M.D., fellow student of Galileo, was graduated from the University of Padua in 1602, he was responsible in his final examination for an hour's discourse on any one of the aphorisms of Hippocrates.

Today many diverse tributes are to be found which are not simply historical in interest, but contemporary, as if Hippocrates held the answers to some of our urgent problems. A. C. Ivy, medical scientist and educator, has this to say:

"Though I had been in medicine for thirty years, I realized for the first time at the Nurnberg trials the full meaning of the contributions of Hippocrates and his school to scientific and technical philosophy of medicine could not survive through the ages unless it was associated with a sound moral philosophy. One cannot conceive of a sound society with medicine that does not have a sound moral philosophy."

Again, an astute observer and practitioner of medicine, Bernard Aschner, has written, "Today Hippocratism is still the worshiped ideal of educated physicians. But during the last hundred years it has remained more or less lip-service." An actively practicing physician, he indicts modern medicine in these terms:

"Through the whole history of medicine there runs, like a bright thread, a more or less permanent struggle between two principal tendencies— empiricism and rationalism. The former, or empirical trend, lays its emphasis on helping and the cure of the sick. The latter, or rationalistic trend, lays its main emphasis on 'scientific' explanations for the causes of disease and the methods of treatment.

He continues:

"Today we are living once more in such an era of extreme intolerant rationalism. We can see the displacement of simple, valuable—nay, fundamental and indispensable—traditional methods of healing in favor of a more sophisticated, theorizing, experimental and technical trend, guided by an exaggerated application of such auxiliary sciences as physics, chemistry and physiology. This trend has even gone so far that established clinical experience has been replaced by the (neorationalism) of natural science."

He further observes:

"Nor is this state of affairs a mere academic proposition, since it influences decisively the fate of the sick. . . . Moreover, our up-to-date medicine is wavering between the therapeutic nihilism of internal medicine and a too-far-reaching operative radicalism in the surgical branches."

He asks for a return to Hippocratic principles.

A third tribute indicating an additional dimension of Hippocrates' message for us was expressed by the present writer at a recent convocation for medical students and faculty members:

"Hippocrates, the Father of Medicine, knew thoroughly that humanistic studies and piety in a physician were not a substitute for technical knowledge. But as a leading educator, he also knew, as few do today, that the intimate and complex relationship between one human being, the physician, and another human being, his sick charge, necessitated something above and beyond, something more inclusive and comprehensive than the pinning on of disease labels, and the execution of their attached medical and surgical recipes. This comprehension is manifest throughout his works in his persistent concern for what pertains to the whole of the patient. He would have been aghast at the notion that the newest of our specialties is psychosomatic medicine, that the patient ever could have been thought of as anything other than a person, an inseparable unit of *psyche* and *soma!* He would have held with St. Thomas (against the Cartesian duality that pervades contemporary thought) that 'since the soul is united to the body as its form, it must necessarily be in the whole body, and in each part thereof.' "

As we have seen, there is professional witness to Hippocrates' capacity for making contributions of perennial value. We also have another type of witness—perhaps a more provocative type. This is the witness of a public as it reflects and cogitates on its collective experience. The testimony is negative; it arises from a sense of disharmony or disruption, an awareness of a deficiency or hidden hunger that permeates our seemingly robust present-day medicine. To bring these thoughts into sharper focus, to evoke any latent discontent with contemporary medicine should prove valuable in a true appreciation of Hippocrates, especially when one reads the works of the father of medicine. All readers of Hippocrates are patients, potential or actual. They should be concerned with medical tradition, for they are the ultimate gainers or losers.

Furthermore, the more vivid the critical insights that arise from one's reflections, the better the background for a reading of Hippocrates. And vividness, like a cure, often can be best achieved by highlighting the defects rather than the assets in the backdrop of our living experiences. Everyone applauds the rescue of men and women from premature death and the sharp reduction in mortality rates which modern medicine has achieved. But even these accomplishments make more manifest the anxieties and morbidities of the living. Let us view, then, the panorama of modern medical practice and sharpen our vision by characterizing— or caricaturing, as the case may be—the dissatisfactions we feel.

We see patients' stomachs turned into apothecaries' crucibles, and the patients perversely enjoying it; the substitution of varishaped and varicolored pills for knife-and-fork nutriments—the tasteless for the tasteful; the push-button electric shock-therapy approach to the psychiatric manifestations of our age; neurosurgeons competitively solving personality difficulties by whittling away irreplaceable brain tissues. We see surgeons displaying their skills in removing so-called nonvital organs, and an increase of medical literature on iatrogenic illnesses.

We witness the growth of highly technical assembly-line medical centers; the disappearance of the humanly sensitive person—the family physician— and his replacement by the automaton concentrating on the mechanically sensitive X ray, electrocardiography and laboratory procedures; complexities of treatment substituting for simplicities, for no other reason than that they are complex and duly impress physicians and patients alike; overspecialization and the consequent decline of the general practitioner; the false separation of the patient's ailment from the ecological environment of home, work and human association.

Finally, we see the veterinarian approach replacing the anthropomorphic approach, with growing confusion as to man's dignity and destiny; the perverse transmuting of normalties into abnormalities. as in obstetrics and pediatrics, and, in general, the over-all substitution of scientism for nature's norms and goals.

Confronted with such a picture, we suspect, to borrow a phrase from T. S. Eliot, that today we have answers for everything but exact ideas about nothing.

Modern Man Over-stimulated and Fearful

Our insensitivity to tradition and its wisdom is not without effect. It gives us modern man, who goes through life with fear of death; who, fearing death, expends his health in hypochondriacal distress; who becomes a vitamin-taking, antacid-consuming, barbiturate-sedated, aspirin-alleviated, weed-habituated, alcohol-inebriated, benzedrine-stimulated, psychosomatically diseased, surgically despoiled animal. Nature's highest product becomes a fatigued, peptic-ulcerated, depressed, sleepless, headachy, nicotinized, overstimulated, neurotic, tonsilless creature.

The reader can judge best to what extent such a characterization is a caricature. In any case, it should heighten our sensibility and increase our docility to Galen's warning that, though we praise Hippocrates, we do not read him or do not understand him or do not put his principles into practice. Reading Hippocrates may reward us with unexpected and needed insights.

In an age when patients markedly dictate the forms of medical practice, there is a certain appropriateness in the fact that Galen was speaking to laymen as well as physicians. The Hippocratic physician recognized the need for the layman to be educated. And, as Jaeger has shown, Hippocratic thought on this matter played a major if not a decisive role in establishing as a basis for the cultural pattern of Greek life the notion of the liberally educated person. His concept of man as being free when he is liberated by the "library" of the liberal arts received its fullest expression in later Greek thought. Aristotle definitively voices it in the opening paragraph of his biological work *Parts of Animals,* where he states that "every inquiry ... the humblest and the noblest alike, seems to admit of two distinct kinds of proficiency; one of which may properly be called scientific knowledge of the subject, while the other is a kind of educational acquaintance with it. For an educated man should be able to form a fair off-hand judgment as to the goodness or badness of the method used by a professor in his exposition." That this is to include medicine is corroborated by his reference in the *Politics* to the three kinds of "physician": ". . . the ordinary physician, the physician of the higher class (the medical scientist), and thirdly, the intelligent man who has studied the art, to whom we attribute the power of judging quite as much as to the professors of the art."

This cultural pattern, so profoundly crystallized by the Hippocratic school, arose not from a preoccupation with disease but from a concern for optimum health. In their hands, medicine was freed from the domination of the demonstrative sciences, such as mathematics and natural science, and was the first discipline of a practical nature to become precisely formulated as such. As a consequence, medicine became the exemplar for other practical sciences, such as ethics and politics. Much of our insight into the Greek concept of medicine comes indirectly from the analogies that were drawn to it, especially by Plato and Aristotle, to clarify less familiar notions in other fields.

Thus, in the *Politics,* Aristotle, when classifying the medically educated

layman with the practicing physician and the medical scientist, is trying
to show the relationship of the electorate to the statesman and the political
scientist. He concludes that the electorate, like the medically educated
layman, the "user," so to speak, may "turn out to be a better judge" than
the others.

We have from the Hippocratic school varied works, prepared for public
discussion, on the nature of disease (e.g., "On The Nature of Man," "The
Sacred Disease") and, at a more practical level, on things similar to present-
day texts in personal hygiene (e.g., "Regimen in Health").

It would be sheer naïveté to think that these and other Hippocratic
works spell out complete answers for us. They are not a true-or-false
compendium in the modern manner. They suffer the handicaps of having
to be translated from a terse and ancient language. They will be in part
obscure, with an aphoristic obscurity not unlike that of metaphysical
poetry. They will communicate through the flux of a past age much
that is strange and foreign to us who are enmeshed in our contingencies.
Finally, Hippocrates will come to us in a corpus diversified in time and
authorship, with some parts duplicated, some parts missing, and some
parts contradicting one another but achieving a wholeness through a
living catechetical and functioning tradition. Thus, we should not expect
an expository work form-fitted to a Great Books audience of the latter half
of the twentieth century.

Hippocrates' Wisdom Eternal

On the other hand, we do start with a common bond: the reality of
man and nature and deity, and the eternal problems of a rational, social,
divinely inspired animal, with his love of life and his capacity for health,
with his subjection to disease, disorder and even irrationality, who is also
unfortunately a money-paying animal. Our effort must be to take from
the father of medicine (who like all fathers has the perspective that comes
from looking both backward and forward) that wisdom which is common
to all ages.

Unfortunately, the wisdom that can be found in Hippocrates is not
foolproof. After we have recovered from the initial surprise of discovering
that the first essay of the father of medicine is entitled *Ancient Medicine,*
we must not make the mistake of thinking that our function as a reader
is simply and smugly to look backward at former errors as if they were
buried once and for all. On the contrary, we must look forward with him.
For, no matter how well they are embalmed, the errors of physicians,

unlike their patients, will be resurrected frequently—by later physicians. Actually we will discover in this essay and in other writings of his school that medicine which was ancient to Hippocrates possessed truths that medicine contemporary to him had lost because of the scientism of the day. If we are astute we will pluck the parallel that Hippocratic medicine, ancient to us, possesses truths that medicine, contemporary to us, has lost through a 'similar scientism.

What wisdom did the father of medicine possess that we, perhaps, lack? In the most general terms we may state that the Hippocratic physician would have had the opportunity of acquiring an active *philosophy* of medicine. This philosophy would give him an understanding of the ends of medicine, of the nature of medicine, of the nature of health and disease, of the nature of the medical act. Furthermore, it would give him a comprehension of the nature of the man who possesses health and disease and the realization that health is not man's ultimate end.

Again, he would be habituated in the attributes necessary to the physician as the maker of health. First, he would be clear in his obligations as a human being living in society. This would demand a liberal education. He would have to know metaphysics and theology in the manner of an educated man, because man has being and a divine goal. He would have to know natural science, because human beings are interconnected with all nature. He would have to be a moralist, possessing a practical knowledge of ethics and knowing how virtue operates among men. He would have to be educated in politics to know his functions and obligations in a society.

Second, he would be habituated in the attributes that belong to him as a physician working for the common good through a particular profession. He would have to be the kind of natural scientist who knows his science as serving an artistic end; he must know nature not simply for the sake of possessing truths about optimum health. He would be a medical artist, for he must have the habit of right reason in respect to making health in cooperation with nature, the exemplar of medical artists. He would have medical experience so that he could recognize that to which he is to apply right reason. He would have prudence or practical wisdom so that he might have right reason in respect to the fitness of his medical acts, which are also human acts.

Finally, he would be able to communicate, for he is not a veterinarian dealing with dumb animals; he must possess his art in an intelligible and communicable way and thus be a rhetorician.

The Hippocratic Oath conveys and epitomizes some of the more general relationships and reveals a series of obligations: to the deities, to the teacher, to the Art (to cure, to conform to its ends, to harm not), to the patient as patient, to the patient as human being, and finally to the physician himself.

Hippocratic Aphorisms Deserve Study

In more specific terms, there are endless facets to be explored and understood, especially as they illuminate the shadows of medical education and practice. That these facets seem inexhaustible testifies to the greatness of these works of the Hippocratic school. The reader will have the opportunity to discover some of them for himself. In passing, perhaps a few should be emphasized and commented upon briefly.

Here, then, are some propositions and prescriptions the writer finds in the Hippocratic school of medicine:

The practice of medicine can never be a science: medicine is an art, having a good to achieve, not a truth to possess. The final goal is the cure, not the diagnosis. Better a cured patient with no diagnosis than an autopsied patient with an exact diagnosis. There may be much intellectual confusion associated with the surgical or medical act; an exciting research experiment for the physician may be an experience of suffering for the patient; and the beautiful pathology found in a patient is hardly such to the person. The physician clearly must separate his scientific instincts from his artistic obligations. Perhaps this would be accelerated if he had to pay rather than render a fee when he sacrificed artistic obligations to satisfy scientific instincts.

The art of medicine cooperates with and mutates nature. It does for nature what nature would do for itself if it could. Hippocrates observes, "though physicians take many things in hand, many diseases are also overcome for them spontaneously. . . . .The gods are the real physicians, though people do not think so." *(Decorum 6.)* Thus, it may be better to do nothing— which requires more thinking but creates less of an impression—than to do something—which frequently requires less thinking but creates a greater impression. There would be agreement with Benjamin Franklin's observation that there is a great deal of difference between a good physician and a bad physician, but very little difference between a good physician and no physician at all. There would also be agreement with Oliver Wendell Holmes's observation that a pair of substantial mammary glands are more advantageous than the two hemispheres of the most learned professor's brain in compounding a nutritive fluid for infants.

A patient cannot be known adequately apart from his environment.
There are many diseases in which one house call is frequently worth more diagnostically than two weeks at a leading medical center. The modern hospital-centered training of a physician is oblivious to this fact. Its narrow approach can well be contrasted with the wider approaches exemplified in part in the opening section of *Airs, Waters, Places.*

The positive production of optimum health, not the cultivation of the hypochondriacal is the ultimate goal in medicine. To borrow from the Greeks, the problem is not to educate diseases but to graduate them into health; not to nurse the real or imaginary diseases along (as in the abuse of bed rest) and encourage their presence as if every person should be a patient till he dies, struggling to old age through the modern extension of the ancient "invention of a lingering death." Hippocrates would have been puzzled at the amounts of patent and prescribed medicine consumed by the public today. He would be amused to observe that self-medication seems to increase in proportion to newspaper, periodical and radio concentration on bodily ills, as in the United States, and that prescribed medicine disproportionately increases with economic accessibility of physicians and druggists, as witnessed in England in recent years.

Health education is ordered toward health and not toward morbid preoccupation with disease. One out of five dies of cancer, we hear. Lesser health organizations find that one out of ten dies of lesser diseases. The fact is that one out of one dies of something. And so we worry about what we do not have, while we do nothing about what we do have; whereas, if we did something about what we do have, we might not develop what we don't have. This is the state of affairs, for instance, in obesity, which is our most prevalent abnormality and which predisposes to all chronic diseases and cancer.

The proper order of treatment is, first, regimen, the medication and lastly, surgery. Regimen for Hippocrates took in the entire dimension of one's habits of life: eating, working, resting, exercising, massaging, sleeping. On the whole, it called for active cooperation in the cure on the part of the patient and not simply for passive participation or resignation. One may contrast the current tendency to the reverse order of treatment, which is epitomized by the fact of a disproportionately high fee paid the surgeon. It is not unrelated to the worship of the hand-minded, the somatic and the material in modern society. Regimen was also ordered to what today is most neglected, positive health. The purpose of regimen here was twofold: a perfective part which attempted to promote optimum health in time

15

present, which was interrelated with a preventive part to protect against disease in the future.

We treat an individual, not a universal. Our diagnostic and prognostic considerations should be based on individuating characteristics which will lead to an individuated therapeusis, not to a routine procedure nor one in which the patient is used as a target for the physician's armamentarium.

Clinical observations should be exact and not colored by our preconceptions; conclusions should record mistakes. Since we learn from mistakes, we should not overemphasize successes, which are frequently short-range and apparent. ". . . those things also give good instruction which after trial show themselves failures and show why they failed." *(On Joints, 47.) Epidemics,* which introduced the concept of an accurate case history and recorded more deaths than cures, should therefore remain a model for us.

The true physician will suffer from the ignorance and stylish therapies of others. "For they praise what seems outlandish before they know whether it is good, rather than the customary which they already know to be good; the bizarre rather than the obvious." *(On Wounds of the Head,* 1.)

Medicine is a profession; as such it becomes the measure of the physician's work and fee. A basic understanding of a professional fee (hardly touched upon in the modern medical school) needs "our consideration as it contributes somewhat to the whole." The following two passages from Hippocrates speak for themselves:

"So one must not he anxious about fixing a fee. For I consider such a worry to be harmful to a troubled patient, particularly if the disease be acute. For the quickness of the disease, offering no opportunity for turning back, spurs on the good physician not to seek his profit but rather to lay hold on reputation. Therefore it is better to reproach patient you have saved than to extort money from those who are at death's door."- *(Precepts,* 4.)

"And if there is an opportunity of serving one who is a stranger in financial straits, give full assistance to all such. For where there is love of man, there is also love of art. For some patients, though conscious that their condition is perilous, recover their health simply through their contentment with the goodness of the physician" - *(Precepts, 6.)*

Judeo-Christian Tradition Enriches Hippocrates

But Hippocrates was a pagan and we may examine, in conclusion, the loss to a physician that results from the absence of the Judeo-Christian tradition. Certainly Hippocrates could have no fundamental awareness of our intrinsic disharmony or of the cause amid cure of the underlying spiritual disorder. Though "where there is love of man, there is also love of the art," the man we love may easily turn out to be ourselves. Love of ourselves, against which the pagan had incomplete immunity, has a diabolical way of interfering with love of man and thus with love of the art. In redirecting love to its highest object, St. Luke, the Patron of Physicians, elevates medicine and so completes and perfects Hippocrates in the manner of grace perfecting nature. St. Luke signifies much for the physician striving for cure (which in its derivation means "care"), and through the physician much for the patient hungering for a care proportionate to his human worth amid destiny.

We must remember, however, that grace acts only through nature. Grace does not replace nor dispense with nature. Grace subsists in and elevates nature. Hippocrates did a profound job of reading the Book of Nature, that book which, St. Thomas says, "God, like a good teacher, has taken care to compose [for us—along with the Book of Holy Scriptures] - - - that we may be instructed in all perfection." Thus St. Thomas, who declares that in this Book of Nature there are "many excellent writings which deliver the truth without falsehood. Wherefore Aristotle, when asked whence it was that he had his admirable learning, replied: 'From things, which do not know how to lie.' " *(Sermo V in Dom. 2 de Adventu.)* Hippocrates could have answered similarly.

We can best appreciate the worth of Hippocrates by considering modern medical schools in this connection. They purport to give their students an integrated medical education, but fail to achieve this comprehensive grasp of nature and fail to realize its prior and basic necessity. The fact is, they are essentially technical schools rather than professional schools. This makes it difficult for them to deal with nature adequately. As a result, the catalytic forces of the Judeo-Christian tradition have little to catalyze. What little they do in this direction is more anatomic than physiologic and more divisive than reparative. Furthermore, they add the tradition of St. Luke to medicine as though they were transplanting a baptized appendix to an unbaptized body. They hardly know that, in many instances, their body is not living but dead. Therefore, in a choice between the pagan medicine of Hippocrates and contemporary medicine—amid we may remember here that the natural law is implanted in the hearts of all men—there is reason to believe that Hippocrates comes closer to God in his vision of medicine than do those myopic ones who miss nature or muddle the application of a God-given tradition.

Medical educators with an insensitivity to the Hippocratic tradition and an insensitivity to the Judeo—Christian tradition miss truth, therefore, in a twofold way. They fail to ascend *to* the 'wholeness of nature's teaching which, comes from a comprehensive understanding of the patient, the physician, and the Art; and they fail to descend *with* wholeness of God's teaching into nature and the concrete world. They narrow the teachings of nature and they narrow the teachings of God.

As a result, in these modern times we are becoming more and more of a paying animal and less and less of a praying animal, as if health were a commodity that could be bought rather than a state which should he sought, not alone through the ministerial functions of the physician but through a wise accommodation of one's nature to nature, and a loving subjection of one's being to God.

Hippocrates is a major step on the road back to a fully integrated and properly humanized medicine and is a prime example of one type of contribution of the Great Books to modern culture and society.

CHAPTER 3

THE INDISPENSABILITY OF HIPPOCRATES

By

John Brehany, PhD

This is the year 2007, almost 2500 years since Hippocrates, known as the Father of Medicine was born. You all recognize his name, but why should you care about the Oath that is attributed to him and the tradition in medicine he inspired? I want to argue that you should care — that it is critical to your satisfaction and your survival as physicians. By the end of my talk, I hope you will come to see the Hippocratic Oath and Tradition as not only indispensable, but inspiring as well. Before I explain what I mean about satisfaction and survival, I will briefly note what the Hippocratic Oath and tradition are not (because sometimes people associate the wrong things with them) and then give you my working definition of what they are and why they are indispensable.

First, a great number of medical schools encourage their students to take some kind of oath; however, most do not take the Hippocratic Oath. In fact, only one school employs the actual Oath attributed to Hippocrates; about half use an abridged or edited version of this and the rest use oaths unrelated to the Hippocratic Oath.[1] Here is the original Hippocratic Oath (Edelstein trans.):[2]

> I swear by Apollo Physician and Asclepius and Hygieia and Panaceia and all the gods and goddesses, making them my witnesses, that I will fulfill according to my ability and judgment this oath and this covenant:

> To hold him who has taught me this art as equal to my parents and to live my life in partnership with him, and if he is in need of money to give him a share of mine, and to regard his offspring as equal to my brothers in male lineage and to teach them this art - if they desire to learn it - without fee and covenant; to give a share of precepts and oral instruction and all the other learning to my sons and to the sons of him who has instructed me and to pupils who have signed the covenant and have taken an oath according to the medical law, but no one else.

> I will apply dietetic measures for the benefit of the sick according to my ability and judgment; I will keep them from harm and injustice.

> I will neither give a deadly drug to anybody who asked for it, nor will I make a suggestion to this effect. Similarly I will not give to a woman an abortive remedy. In purity and holiness I will guard my life and my art.

> I will not use the knife, not even on sufferers from stone, but will withdraw in favor of such men as are engaged in this work.

> Whatever houses I may visit, I will come for the benefit of the sick, remaining free of all intentional injustice, of all mischief and in

---

1   Orr Robert, Pang Norman, Pellegrino Edmund, and Siegler Mark. Use of the Hippocratic Oath: A review of twentieth century practice and a content analysis of oaths, administered in Medical Schools in the U.S. and Canada in 1993. J Clin. Ethics, 8:377-388,1997

2   Edelstein, Ludwig. "The Hippocratic Oath; Text, Translation and Interpretation," in Ancient Medicine: Selected Papers of Ludwig Edelstein. O. Temkin and C.L. Temkin, eds. (Baltimore, MD: Johns Hopkins Press, 1967),pp 3-63.

particular of sexual relations with both female and male persons, be they free or slaves.

What I may see or hear in the course of the treatment or even outside of the treatment in regard to the life of men, which on no account one must spread abroad, I will keep to myself, holding such things shameful to be spoken about.

If I fulfill this oath and do not violate it, may it be granted to me to enjoy life and art, being honored with fame among all men for all time to come; if I transgress it and swear falsely, may the opposite of all this be my lot.

Second, the Hippocratic Tradition is not synonymous with "ancient medicine" or even "traditional medicine" — if by those terms you mean "how medicine used to be practiced either 2000 years ago or 200 years ago — in short, any time before the mid-20th century. In particular, the Hippocratic Tradition should not be identified with the image of the physician in America in the 1950s (perhaps the zenith of the awe with which physicians were viewed). That status and image, however impressive, were constructed over the course of a century.[3] It was comprised of many good elements, but some problematic elements as well. Moreover, this status and image were not always enjoyed by physicians across time and cultures.

In a nutshell, the Hippocratic Tradition is a disciplined approach to medicine based upon the values expressed in the Hippocratic Oath and a rational approach to the healing art of medicine. By a "rational approach" to medicine, I mean an approach in which reason triumphs over ideology. The rational character of Hippocratic medicine became evident in the ancient world when it broke from the then popular mold of seeking supernatural explanations for human illness and, more importantly, because it rejected the notion that the power of medicine could be applied either to heal or to kill. In the 20th century there have been several ideologies — organized agendas of ideas and values (such as those found in the Nazi and Soviet totalitarian systems) — that have tried to define the enterprise of medicine. Whether by subordinating medicine to the power or projects of the nation-state or to the goal of achieving wealth, status or power, these ideologies

3   Starr, P. The Social Transformation of American Health Care. Basic Books, 1982.

chose something outside the terms of health and healing to define the rules and goals of medicine. In the Hippocratic (reasoned) approach to medicine, rational inquiry is focused on understanding the nature of health and the causes of disease, and the power of healing is viewed, not as existing for the benefit of the physician or the state, but for the benefit of the patient.

What are Hippocratic values? I suggest that three fundamental values can be found in the Hippocratic Oath: First, the belief that the physician's power is a limited power — limited by the divine (either the gods referenced by the Oath or the One God shared by the sons of Abraham) as well as by the fundamental good of human life (which the Oath forswears acting directly against in proscribing physician-assisted suicide and abortion). Second, the good of loyalty and service to the medical profession itself— which should not be identified either with professional courtesy or clannishness. Rather, the Hippocratic physician realizes that medicine as an art can only be learned and practiced in a disciplined community that shares certain values and hands on a shared practice from generation to generation. And third, that the healing mission of the physician is a work undertaken in fundamental concert with nature and, above all, with respect for the well-being of the patient. This third value can be seen in the reference to the use of dietetic measures, in the rejection of surgery, and in the rejection of all abuses of power regarding the patient and his/her family.

Why are these values in the Hippocratic Oath significant? One way of explaining this is to acknowledge Leon Kass's point[4] that the Hippocratic Oath is the best distillation yet of the core essence of medicine. Medicine will always be shaped by the times and places in which it is practiced, but the core tasks and relationships that give rise to the physician-patient relationship — a person in need of healing and a person dedicated to the science and art of that vocation -- remain and always will.[5] An interesting lens through which to view both these core tasks of medicine and the social forces that shape the practice of medicine is to compare some influential Oaths and Codes of Ethics that have existed over time. I think you would find it very interesting to compare the Oath of Hippocrates with the Code of Ethics of the AMA[6] from 1847, or the Oath of Soviet Physicians,[7] 1971

4   Kass, L. "Is there a medical ethic" in Toward a More Natural Science. Free Press, New York, NY, 1985. pp 224-246.
5   Pellegrino E, and Thomasma. A Philosophical Basis of Medical Practice. Oxford University Press, New York, NY, p.81, 1987.
6   Code of Ethics of the AMA, 1947.
7   Oath of Soviet Physician. (1971). Encyclopedia of Bioethics. Appendix, p

with the Solemn Oath of a Physician of Russia,[8] 1992. What you would clearly see in comparing either of these pairs is that one (Hippocratic Oath or Solemn Oath of a Physician of Russia) is defined above all in terms of the values inherent in medicine while the other (Code of Ethics of the AMA or the Oath of Soviet Physicians) is defined by the broader social values of their place and time.

But this is not merely a nice point to acknowledge; I propose that it is a necessary point to understand; necessary for two things: (1) for keeping your perspective; and (2) for keeping your profession. What do I mean?

I. <u>Keeping your perspective</u>. Keeping your perspective is key to your satisfaction as physicians. I don't think this is a truism. The practice of medicine is more complicated than ever before. It is not primarily that there are new diseases to deal with (although there are now 30 STIs as compared with 3 in 1960). Rather, it is that there are an always growing number of technologies and medicines to treat human illness and injuries. But not only this. There are also new laws and regulations designed to control the power of physicians and legions of codes, rules and software designed to control reimbursement for medical services. Each one of these new areas is complex, challenging, and ever-changing. It is now common for physicians to complain that they spend more time on the telephone arguing with insurance reps or doing paperwork than they do seeing patients. It is demonstrable that the threat of lawsuits affects clinical judgment, causing physicians to practice "defensive medicine." And the role of government in paying for health care services continues to grow.

A physician cannot afford to ignore or even to pay half-hearted attention to these features of modem medical practice. But even if he or she fulfilled every law, dotted every "I," etc., this would not mean that he/she is a good physician, and it would not make him/her a fulfilled physician. Rather, only if, in addition to covering these requisite bases, a physician remains rooted in and shaped by a Hippocratic approach to medicine, can he/she be described as a good physician, and can he/she have a chance of attaining a deep and lasting satisfaction.

2. <u>Keeping your profession</u>. Remaining rooted in Hippocratic vision and values is not only a matter of satisfaction; it is a matter of professional survival. It is essential for individual and professional integrity. A big claim; why is it so?

2690.

8   Oath of the Physicians of Russia. (1992). Encyclopedia of Bioethics. Appendix, p2690.

In short, because in any human community or endeavor, there are both a number of the individuals involved and a range of diverse goods served. Something must hold the whole system together. There must be a "key" both for establishing priorities and for resolving conflicts, etc.

Here is a maxim from physics that has some applicability to sociology, including the practice of medicine in society — "nature abhors a vacuum." Something will always rush into to fill the void. Someone and some values must supply the key to ordering priorities, establishing rules and standards, and resolving conflicts. The question is, who will constitute that authority—for the medical profession as a whole or in the physician-patient relationship, and where will the values come from? Will the authority be legislators, bureaucrats, lawyers, judges, activists, etc.? What values will rule — will they come from the law, regulatory requirements, market demand, "customer satisfaction," or budgetary considerations and constraints? If physicians are not able to create a profession in which the authentic goods of healing are discerned, affirmed, and served, then medicine will become a tool of some other system and subject to its values and standards. Ironically, precisely because medicine serves such fundamental human goods, it is all the more tempting for people to use it for their own ends and for other institutions to try to control it.

As much as I think it is important to note these dangers, I don't want to make the Hippocratic Oath and Tradition sound like a defensive strategy. I think they are better described as a positive and guiding resource for you in your career as physicians. As I noted before, the vocation and tasks of medicine have not changed, even though the tools, institutions, and social settings in which medicine is practiced have changed profoundly. I think it is also fair to say that the temptations of those who practice medicine (to achieve wealth, status or control, or to give people what they demand rather than what they need, to name only a few) also have not changed. The Hippocratic Oath and Tradition will empower you not merely because you have read about them or even memorized the Oath. They will empower you to the extent that they shape how you view your identity and your work as physicians.

Understanding, interpreting and implementing the values of the Hippocratic Oath and Tradition is not something that can be achieved in medical school or even at the end of medical residency. It is a process that takes years. I hope this short talk, and the discussion that we are about to have, will inspire you to begin this process if you have not already.

CHAPTER 4

A PHILOSOPHICAL BASIS FOR THE PATIENT-PHYSICIAN INTERACTION

By

Edmund Pellegrino, MD

The Fact of Illness

Medicine and physicians exist because humans become ill. Illness is a subjective state, one in which a human being detects some change, acute or chronic, in his/her mode of existence based in anxiety about the functions of body or mind. Illness may or may not be associated with demonstrable pathology. What is crucial to being ill is the perception of an altered state of existence, one in which the patient interprets some symptom or sign as an indication that he/she is no longer "healthy," according to the patient's own definition of that fluid and multi-interpretable word.

A person who arrives at the conclusion that he/she is "ill" becomes a patient—one who bears some disability, some deficiency or concern, one who is no longer "whole," one who perceives special limits on his or her accustomed activity.

The person who becomes a patient suffers what is nothing less than an ontological assault. In our usual state we see ourselves identified with our bodies, facing the world and acting on it in essential unity. In illness the body is interposed between us and reality—it impedes our choices and actions and is no longer fully responsive. The body stands opposite to the self. Instead of serving us, we must serve it. It intrudes on our existence rather than enhancing or enriching it. We can no longer use it for transbodily purposes.

With this assault on the ontological unity of body and self, illness erodes the image we have fashioned of ourselves over the years. That image harmonizes our deficiencies and our strong points; we carefully and laboriously protect and refurbish it; we delicately balance it against the external exigencies of human life. Illness forces a reappraisal and that poses a threat to the old image; it opens up all the old anxieties and imposes new ones––often including the real threat of death or drastic alterations in lifestyle. This ontological assault is aggravated by the loss of most of the freedoms we identify as peculiarly human. The patient is no longer free to make rational choices among alternatives. He lacks the knowledge and the skills necessary to cure himself or gain relief of pain and suffering. In many illnesses, the patient is not even free to reject medicine, as in severe trauma or other over-whelming acute emergencies. Voluntarily or not, the patient is forced to place himself under the power of another person, the health professional, who has the knowledge and the skills which can heal–but also harm. This involuntary need grounds the axiom of vulnerability from which follows the obligations of the physician.

When a person becomes "ill," therefore in an exceptionally vulnerable state, one which severely compromises his customary human freedoms to use his body for transbodily purposes, to make his own decisions, to act for himself, and to accept or reject the services of others. The state of being ill is therefore a state of "wounded humanity," of a person compromised in his fundamental capacity to deal with his vulnerability.

How unique is the state of illness? Is not vulnerability a common condition in many other human situations? After all, the prisoner is deprived of freedom and civil rights; the poor and the socially outcast are constrained even in the most mundane matters of life; none of us is totally "free"; we must all conform to some set of social conventions. But in none of these situations is our capacity to deal with our vulnerability so impaired as in illness. We feel, usually, that we can cope with almost all of the other states of vulnerability if we have our "health." After all, we perceive health as a means toward freedom and other primary values. We ask only to be released from prison, given a job or money, and if we are healthy, we can rebuild our humanity and the integrity of our person. In illness, none of these things will help. Our essential mechanisms for coping with all other existential exigencies are compromised; we face the threat of loss of life itself, or we are suddenly asked to live a life which appears not worth living.

There is, therefore, a special dimension of anguish in illness. That is why healing cannot be classified as a commodity, or as a service on a par with going to a mechanic to have one's car fixed, to a lawyer for repair of one's legal fences, or even to a teacher for repair of one's defects in knowledge. The teacher-student, lawyer-client, serviceman-customer relationships have some of the elements of the physician-patient relationship. There is in them an inequality of knowledge and skill, and one person seeks assistance from another who professes to provide it. What is different is the unique ontological assault of illness on the body-self unity, and the primacy of the freedom to deal with all other life situations which illness removed. Without denying the analogy with, let us say, the lawyer-client relationship, it would be difficult to argue that the degree of injury to our humanity and the kind of injury we suffer in litigation are identical in their existential consequences to being ill.

The Act of Profession

In the presence of a patient in the peculiar state of vulnerable humanity which is illness, the health professional makes a "profession." He or she "declares aloud" that he has special knowledge and skills, that he can heal, or help, and that he will do so in the patient's interest, not his own. According to the *Oxford English Dictionary*, the etymology of the word "profession"–from the verb *profiteri*, to declare aloud or publicly–is closer to the meaning of the act than more recent formulations. That is what entering a profession means–not simply becoming a member of a defined group with a common education, standards of performance, and a common ethic. These are all secondary conditions of the central act of profession, which is an active, conscious declaration, voluntarily entered into and signifying willingness to assume the obligations necessary to make the declaration authentic.

All health professionals make this act of profession publicly when they accept a degree at graduation, when they take the oath of their profession, and, most important, every time they present themselves to a patient in need who seeks their assistance in healing. They make the act of profession implicitly, but nonetheless undeniably. The expectation is thus induced in the ill person that the declaration will be true and authentic, that the professional's knowledge and skill are genuine, and that the professional's concern for the patient's interests will be truly exercised.

Medicine is, of course, not alone in making an act of profession which invites specific expectations of performance. Lawyers, teachers, and ministers similarly declare a special competence and its use in the interests of those who seek their aid. Their clients also lack something they need. Like the patient, they too are vulnerable to varying degrees. The ethics of each profession rests on the authenticity of its claim–the physician's claim to restore health, the lawyer's to seek justice, the teacher's to redress ignorance, and the minister's to teach the way of salvation.

The act of profession is a promise made to another person, who is in need and therefore existentially vulnerable. The relationship between the professional and those he or she serves is characterized by an inequality in which the professional holds the balance of power. All the usual ethical obligations of making and keeping promises apply, but with a difference–the inequality of power poses special obligations on the person who professes. The professional-client relationship is not simply a contract between equals in which each party can negotiate in his own interest, since one part is not free not to negotiate. Medicine, law, teaching, and the ministry do not supply products in the usual legal and commercial sense.

Each profession fulfills the promise inherent in its act of profession by a specific action which identifies that profession. This central act is the vehicle of authenticity and the bridge which joins the need of the one seeking help with the promise of the one professing to help. We can examine that central act only for medicine, though analogous analyses are applicable to other professions.

The Central Act of Medicine
A patient in need who consults a physician wants to know what is wrong, what can be done about it, and what should be done. These three questions, and the subjects of questions which contribute to answering them, taken together constitute the anatomy of clinical judgment previously developed. The final question--what should be done?—is the major focus of the patient's attention and the end toward which the whole process must be directed. It eventuates in a recommended action. While all the other questions leading to it can be reopened, the recommended action is, once taken, irretrievable.

The end of medicine, formally considered, is therefore a right and good healing action taken in the interests of a particular patient. All the science and art of the physician converge on the choice: among the many things that can be done, that which should be done for this person in this particular situation of life. It is a choice of what is right in the sense of what conforms scientifically, logically, and technically to the patient's needs and a choice of what is good, what is "worth- while" for this patient. The recommended action intermingles technical and moral dimensions which may not always be immediately reconcilable.

This culmination in a right and good healing action is what constitutes medicine *qua* medicine. Diagnosis and therapeutics singly and together serve this end. The physician acts as physician only when he particularizes the conclusions about what is wrong and what can be done in a decision about what ought to be, must be, may be, or should not be done for this patient, here and now.

The patient expects the end of medicine to be an action which is right and good for him. This is the promise he perceives in the act of profession, collectively from organized medicine, and singularly from his personal physician or physicians. It is what he expects also from medical and health organizations—the team, the hospital, or the agency.

The medical act combines technical and moral decision making in a way which makes it a moral enterprise of a special kind. Each medical decision involves the complicated interplay of several value sets—those of the physician, of the patient, and of society. In a pluralistic society, these value sets may differ sharply from each other. The possibilities of conflict in the conception of the good between physician and patient are many. A very special problem in medical decision making is how to resolve these conflicts in a morally defensible way.

For the conflicts of values occur in a relationship of inequality inherent in the vulnerability of the patient, as we have outlined it above. The assault of illness on the usual freedoms of the human being presents an immediate and present danger that the patient's values might be violated or that the physician may confuse technical with moral authority. The patient's moral agency is at risk, and a special obligation of the act of profession is to protect that moral agency while treating the patient.

By virtue of his act of profession, the physician raises specific expectations and thus voluntarily assumes certain specific obligations. It is these obligations, as well as those of the patient to the physician, which we shall examine next.

Obligations Arising from the Special Nature of the Patient-Physician Relationship

The obligations which arise from the construal of the patient-physician relationship outlined here could form the philosophical basis for a professional ethic—one which would bind the physician regardless of the position he might take on any of the specific moral dilemmas of medicine. A cursory examination of these obligations can illustrate the primacy of the acts of profession and medicine taken in the face of the fact of illness.

Let it be clear that no new moral principles need be elaborated. The well-adopted moral principles of truth telling and promise keeping, as well as the principles of non-harm and vulnerability, will suffice, but modulated by those special existential circumstances which define the relationship of one needing to be healed confronting one professing to heal. The same principle would apply by analogy to the lawyer client, teacher-student, minister-subject relationships, each modified by the specific expectations generated by the act of profession each makes when a patient or client is confronted seeking assistance.

To begin with, the act of medical profession is inauthentic and a lie unless it fulfills the expectation of technical competence. If the special knowledge upon which the act of profession is based is wanting, then the whole relationship begins with a lie. The decision may even fortuitously turn out to be the "right and good" one for the patient, but if it does, it is based on chance, not knowledge. The patient has been deceived into believing the advice he received is the fruit of the physician's competence. The far greater likelihood is that the incompetent physician will not make the right or good decision. Then he becomes worse than a quack. The latter at least follows a system which makes no claim to being scientific, while the incompetent physician enshrouds his ignorance in a mantle of science.

The moral obligation to be competent is a lifelong one and an affair of daily concern. It begins with a sound medical education and house staff training, and goes on to a dedication to continuing education, a willingness to subject his decisions to peer review, an openness to criticism by one's colleagues, a willingness to confess ignorance or error to the patient, and a concentrated and sustained effort to deepen one's clinical craftsmanship. Competence, then, is a moral imperative, and a clear statement of that fact together with its fullest implications should be an essential element in any professional code. Competence is explicitly required by the first four principles of the latest revision of the AMA code. It is equated therein with "scientific" medicine. Such a formulation is correctly applicable to the technical steps involved in diagnosis, prognosis, and therapeutics. It includes also the art and skill needed to perform the recommended procedures safely and with a minimum of discomfort.

But in the complex anatomy of clinical judgment, competence is a necessary, but not sufficient, condition of a moral medical transaction and an authentic act of profession. Competence must itself be shaped by the end of the medical act–a right and good healing action for a particular patient. Competence must be employed in the best interest of the patient, and wherever possible that interest must conform with the patients values and sense of what it is to be healthy.

Technically correct conclusions may not necessarily be in the patient's best interest when that interest is defined in the patient's terms, for example, abortion for a Catholic, transfusion for a Jehovah's Witness, prolonging life in someone prepared to die, or "letting" another die who wants to live what may seem to the physician an unsatisfying life. A scientifically correct medical conclusion, its "oughtness," can range from "must," "should," "may," "need not," or "must not," depending upon the interacting moral agencies of patient and physician.

The physician has a special moral obligation to assure and facilitate the patient's moral agency, especially in the light of the patient's special vulnerability. To assure a fully participatory moral agency, the physician must repair to the extent possible the wounded humanity and state of inequality of the sick person. He does so only in part by curing, or containing, illness or relieving pain and anxiety. These must be complemented by disclosure of the information necessary for valid choice and genuine consent and by guarding against manipulation of choice and consent to accommodate to the physician's personal or social philosophy of the good life.

A first requirement, therefore, is to remedy the patient's information deficit as completely as possible. Information must be clear and understandable and in the patient's language. He must know the nature of his illness, its prognosis, the alternative modes of treatment, their probable effectiveness, cost, discomfort, side effects, and the quality of life they may yield. Disclosure must include degrees of ignorance as well as knowledge and the physician's own limitations.

The physician who is conscious of the special nature of his act of profession will not easily excuse himself from the obligation of disclosure on the grounds that the patient cannot understand or will be harmed by the information. There are few, if any, evidences that such knowledge is deleterious, the Hippocratic warnings to the contrary. Indeed, in those rare instances where the matter has been studied, informed patients show a lower anxiety and complication rate than the uninformed.

Reducing the inequality in information between patient and physician is essential in obtaining a morally valid consent which is the vehicle for expression of the patient's moral agency. More is required than the minimal conditions of a legally valid consent, which is after all, guarantee against the grosser violations of the patient's right to decide. A morally valid consent moves closer to the realization of both senses of the word "con-sent" (Latin: *consentire*), to feel and to know something together. Patient and physician, therefore, must each feel he knows and understands the available facts, and each must feel he is truly part of the decision making.

When the patient cannot participate in the decision, the physician must deal with the patient's surrogate—the family, guardian, or the court. The obligations to respect the patient's value system are the same. When dealing with surrogates, however, an additional obligation is imposed, and that is to be sure that they do in fact have the patient's interests at heart. In the case of the unconscious patient or the child, the physician must assure himself that the surrogate, parent, or family does not unconsciously wish the patient's demise.

This state of feeling and knowing together places the actual locus of decision making somewhere between physician and patient, and not really with one or the other. As in any relationship between humans, medical or otherwise, obtaining consent requires persuasion, a mutual accommodation of wills. It is extremely difficult to set limits on the degree to which manipulation of consent is morally permissible. It is important for this essay only to indicate that the physician must be alert to those subtle choices of words, nuances of emphasis, or body language which tips the patient's consent in the direction of what the physician feels is "good." It is unrealistic to expect even the most ethically sensitive physician not to wish the patient would make certain choices. In some cases some degree of persuasion may even be ethically obligatory.

No set of rules could encompass all the subtle complexities of even the most ordinary relationship between two persons, much less the special dimensions peculiar to the medical transaction in which one person in special need seeks the assistance of another who professes to help. The morality of clinical judgment goes well beyond the merely technical and scientific probity of the craft.

There are times when the physician can and should exert moral agency for the patient and make the value choice in his behalf. One instance would be when the patient or family request him to do so even after the physician has attempted to provide the necessary information and has taken all pains to be clear and unequivocal about the choices. Some patients and families are either emotionally or educationally ill-equipped to deal with such difficult decisions. They may then ask the physician to "decide." The physician then has a mandate to assume moral agency, and it would be a failure of the authenticity of his act of profession not to say what should be done. The same applies when the situation is of such an urgent nature that to consult the patient or even his or her family would be impossible or would delay emergency treatment. In the operating and emergency rooms, the intensive-care and coronary-care units, the obligations we have stressed must be drastically modified because the patient's interest itself overrides even these fundamental requirements of medical morality. The retrospective examination of how, for what reasons, and according to what value sets the decisions were made is an essential antidote to overzealous assumption of moral authority even in emergency situations.

Here, too, a caveat is in order. For the physician to say simply that he would treat the patient as he would treat himself or a member of his family is morally unsound. This misinterpretation of the golden rule would only reopen the possibility of overriding the patient's wishes. The golden rule in medical decisions is to be observed rather differently: We should so act that we accord the patient the same opportunity to express or actualize his own view of what he considers worthwhile as we would desire for ourselves. This latter interpretation of the golden rule is fully consistent with the view of authenticity of the act of profession we have developed in this essay.

What obligations of this type require is a combination of conscious advertence to the meanings of the three elements—the fact of illness, the act of profession, and the act of medicine—with compassion. We do not think this has to involve the *iatrike philia*, the love of which Pedro Lain-Entralgo speaks as the fundamental link in his superb phenomenological study of the physician-patient relationship. It does require the capacity to "feel with" the patient something of the existential situation he is experiencing in the condition of illness, whether it is somatic or physical in origin. Not to be able to feel something of the patient's anguish and anxiety before the ontological assault of illness is to rely on only a rational adumbration of the obligations which inhere in the act of profession. But even this is superior to the more traditional conception of the physician as benevolent agent of both technical and moral decision making who decides what is "best" for the patient.

Many aspects of the physician's obligations which could be derived from the philosophy of the medical transaction proposed here have not been touched upon. Those chosen are meant to be illustrative, and not comprehensive. We have not discussed, for example, how to resolve conflicts in values between the physician's social and patient responsibilities, the obligations of the profession as a corporate whole, or the applicability of these principles when the physician functions in a collectivity as a member of a team, or an institution.

Also, on this view, there is a set of obligations which would bind the patient so that we can begin to develop an ethics of the "good" patient. If the physician construes his act of profession as a promise of a special kind given under special conditions, and if the patient understands it that way, then the patient incurs certain obligations as well. He must be truthful in the information he gives the physician; he must avoid manipulating the physician in consent; he must follow recommendations mutually agreed upon faithfully; he must educate himself sufficiently to comprehend the facts disclosed to him, and take the trouble to be sure he does understand; he must not consult another physician without informing his medical attendant unless he suspects dishonesty or malpractice. Further, he is partially obligated, by the fact that he is a member of the human race, to participate in reasonable experiments which are either aimed at healing his disease (therapeutic) or at discovering possible cures for this disease for others (nontherapeutic), provided the other rules for professional behavior are followed.

We say "partially obligated" because the vulnerability of the patient excuses him from any absolute obligation.

The principle of autonomy and the principle of partial obligation enunciated above represent almost a classic example of the possible clash between two goods. On the one hand, the person who is ill is clearly given the opportunity and the freedom to attend to his needs for healing, a value which takes precedence over any altruism to be demanded of him. However, the ill person is also a member of the human race and has obligations to help foster the understanding of the disease so that either he or others might benefit.

The patient, in short, in the relationship we have described, owes the physician the same respect for his values and cannot demand that the physician violate them even when the patient might benefit. The patient cannot ask his physician to practice deception with insurance companies and governmental agencies. In sum, even though the vulnerability imposed by illness makes the patient more vulnerable, the tyranny of the patient is as wrong as the tyranny of the physician.

This construal of the patient-physician relationship calls, therefore, for mutual respect and compassion, even though it involves one person who is less free and more vulnerable. That is why the relationship cannot be regarded as a contract or even a covenant. It is not an agreement between two parties more or less equal, more or less free, who can negotiate terms for the delivery of some service or commodity. Medical care is not a commodity one may choose as freely as one chooses automobiles or television sets.

What we propose is a mutually binding set of obligations, predicted upon a special kind of human interaction and deriving its morality from the empirical realities in the relationship which specify it among human relationships. These specifications could be the basis for a philosophically justifiable statement of principles—a code—common to all physicians, indeed to all healers. If their implications are expanded, we can even hope for a more general code applicable to all the health professions at least in part since all health professionals make an act of profession in the sense we have defined it here.

The post-Hippocratic reconstruction of professional ethics is therefore possible. We need not return to the ethics of the good craftsman, as in our Greek beginnings. We can instead extend and build upon the idea of Scribonius Largus and Panaetius that there is an ethic specific to each profession, based in the nature of that profession, and philosophically justifiable.

CONCLUSION

Looked at historically, our line of reasoning has taken us away from the dominant sources of medical morality—that is, the Hippocratic *Corpus* and the oath especially, away from both the craft and privileged-status ethic. My inclination has been, rather, to the extension and elaboration of the idea of profession as it was advanced by Scribonius Largus and Panaetius and the middle Stoics. I have suggested a derivation of medical ethics from the specific relationship of three phenomena of the medical transaction rather than applying philosophical conceptions drawn outside of medicine to medicine. In contra-distinction to Scribonius Largus, I have not made *humanitas* the specific end of medicine, nor as with Lain-Entralgo the *iatrike philia*, but rather a right and good healing action for a particular patient. This is what the physician professes, what the patient expects, and what must be offered in the presence of the state of wounded humanity we call illness. This is the foundation of professional ethics, the source of medical morality, and the leitmotiv of a more satisfactory professional code of how the physician would act *qua* physician. It is necessarily antecedent to whatever position may be taken in specific moral dilemmas. Indeed, sensitively attended to, it assures the morality of the personal transaction even when there is a difference between physician and patient or physician and physician about particular medical moral problems.

CHAPTER 5

MEDICINE AS A MORAL ART: THE HIPPOCRATIC PHILOSOPHY OF HERBERT RATNER, M.D.

By

Patrick G. D. Riley, PhD

From early in his career, Herbert Ratner stood in the forefront of opposition to utilitarian medicine, such as to a state-regulated, commercialized, medicine and—not least—to a merely technological medicine. A physician since 1935, he was founder and editor of the influential quarterly *Child & Family,* and a major contributor to the *Encyclopedia Britannica's* guide to the "Great Books," the *Syntopicon.*

As director of public health for the Chicago suburb of Oak Park, he attracted national attention when he refused to dispense free Salk polio vaccine without explaining its risks to parents. The village board threatened him with dismissal—an example of politicians exercising medical judgment. He was promptly vindicated when on May 8, 1955, the U.S. Health Services suspended distribution of the vaccine for reasons of safety.

Dr. Ratner's critique of the methodology of the supposedly inactivated Salk vaccine, which from 1955 to 1963 contained Simian Virus 40, drew international attention when published in the November, 1955 *Bulletin of the American Association of Public Health Physicians,* of which he was then editor. It was corroborated independently by a study of the West German Health Ministry.

As associate clinical professor of family and community medicine at Loyola University Stritch School of Medicine, Chicago, he helped in the foundation of the La Leche League for the promotion of breast-feeding. He remained a consultant of the League until his death. Nor did Dr. Ratner's work for the family go unnoticed in Rome; in 1982 the Holy See named him a consultor to its Council for the Family.

For Ratner, the strongest protection the medial profession can marshal against the technological temptation and against threats from business, government, and utilitarianism is the Hippocratic Oath, and the Hippocratic philosophy of medicine summed up in the Oath but also found in the writings of the Hippocratic school.

Perhaps it should be said at the outset that Dr. Ratner's hostility to utilitarianism–"the greatest good for the greatest number" at the expense of individual persons—can scarcely be traced to his Jewishness and the role that utilitarian-oriented physicians took in Nazi campaigns against Jews. He was a champion of Hippocratic medicine long before the postwar Nuremberg trials, which revealed how deeply physicians were implicated in Nazi campaigns to kill the unfit, and to subject members of groups deemed inferior to painful and lethal experiments. He found the basis for his Hippocratic philosophy of medicine as a medical student in the '30s, while reading Hippocrates and the great philosopher of nature, Aristotle. They led him to the study of St. Thomas Aquinas, and eventually into the Catholic Church.

The day the *New York Times* lamented commercial restrictions on an abortion-oriented technique, I went to Chicago to celebrate, with an overflow crowd, Dr. Ratner's 90th birthday. I have counted myself a disciple for half a century, from the moment I heard him speak at Catholic University in January 1949, and I probably should make by debt to him clear. His account of the nature of nature, so to speak, and his emphasis on nature as the norm of normality (again so to speak), made an indelible impression. In the intervening decades we became friends, and I continued to learn from him. Like the gift of his friendship, this gift of wisdom is priceless, and the present essay, designed to hand on the wisdom of Herbert

Ratner to others, is an act of piety in the classic sense of an attempt to repay what can never be repaid.

Herbert Ratner's most priceless legacy to a medical profession beset by threats from within and without is a profound explanation of Hippocratic medicine and its implications, pithily and persuasively expressed. No physician armed with this philosophy—a philosophy articulated by Hippocrates and his school, and since supported by thousands of years of productive tradition, a philosophy responsible in large part for the reverence so long and so willingly paid the profession—no physician so armed need search for rebuttals to the philosophically dated and historically discredited utilitarianism that presents itself, now under this guise and now under that, as modernization.

The Hippocratic physician will repudiate with scorn any suggestion that killing is a part of his profession. While even those laymen who know that Dr. Jack Kevorkian is an aberration may have difficulty articulating why, the Hippocratic physician can unmask Kevorkian as no less a traitor to his profession and those under his care than the physicians who sold out to the Nazis: he need only explain what has preserved medicine as a profession for thousands of years, namely its unshakable ethic, summed up in the Hippocratic Oath.

The Oath has not merely summarized this ethic: the Oath has committed the profession to it, and made it its very soul. Moreover—and this is integral to Dr. Ratner's philosophy—medicine became a profession precisely because of the Oath, for in professing it one became a doctor, that is a teacher (as the Oath required of him), and a healer (as the Oath made him swear to be), and none other.

Doctors who abandoned their sworn Oath at the behest of the Nazi regime were subject to the death penalty at the international tribunal in Nuremberg. Had they remained faithful to their sworn word, not only their patients and their profession but their own person would have been protected. The principle holds today: a medical profession permeated with the ethic of Hippocratic Medicine will stand as a rock against the ethically dubious encroachments, indeed against the most brutal bullying, of big finance and big government alike.

As for the technological temptation, how Hippocratic medicine helps doctors resist that takes some explaining.

The governing principle here as throughout Herbert Ratner's philosophy, which is the philosophy of Hippocrates and Aristotle, is nature. Both the morality and the effectiveness of medicine—not excluding the effectiveness of medical technology—hang upon its respect for nature. Ratner sees nature as the healer as well as the norm. No less significantly, he sees nature as the vicar of God's retribution.

> **Plants automatically lead good plant lives (Ratner observes). They do not have the freedom to do otherwise. They are activated by tropisms which determinatively direct them to the good plant life…. It is through these means that plants, though unknowledgeable of the ends, fructify and flourish and attain their ends.**
>
> **Animals other than man also automatically lead good animal lives. They, too, do not have the freedom to do otherwise. They are activated through hierarchized instincts, which reflect the urge of all living things 'to partake in the eternal and divine' in the only way possible to them, by self-propagation.[1]**

There Dr. Ratner is quoting Aristotle.[2] It was Aristotle's perception of the role of purpose in nature, its inner drive toward a goal, that guided not only philosophy but theology and physical science until the seventeenth century, when the spectacular successes of empirical science, which depends on description for its method and on prediction for its justification, dealt the concept of intrinsic natural purpose a blow from which it is still reeling.

That tended to return philosophy and all depending on it to their primitive state in the mists of prehistory. Aristotle, giving us a brief account of philosophy before his time, recalls the pioneer thinkers who tried to explain the world in terms of matter and of mathematics, and thus were precursors of the scientism of the nineteenth century, still palely loitering. "Hence when a man spoke of mind in nature," Aristotle recalled, probably referring to Anaxagoras, "he seemed like a sane man speaking among lunatics."

In Ratner's scheme of things, learning always falls short of the wisdom of nature. Reliance on what empirical science has taught us leads to disaster when our philosophical understanding of nature has not kept pace with our empirical knowledge of nature, and does not undergird it.

---

1   "The Natural Institution of the Family Challenged", *Journal of the North American Montessori Teachers' Association*, Vol. 19, No.2 (Spring 1994), p. 121.

2   *De anima*, II, iv.

Ratner lays the groundwork for this concept in a passage bristling with characteristic paradox:

Man's free choice is not left to itself. Though he is not compelled by tropisms or instincts, man is not left adrift in directing his natural destiny. He has the natural inclinations of a mammalian and social animal.

There are inclinations which in Pascal would correspond to his "simple Pure ignorance." These natural inclinations can be confounded by higher education, which give the illusion of a high order of intellectual and educational development but which, in reality, falls far short of Pascal's "learned ignorance. ...As we have nouveaux riches, so we have nouveaux intellectuals. Such people have been educated out of their "simple pure ignorance" but unfortunately have not been educated into a "learned ignorance."[3]

Pascal's "learned ignorance," in Ratner's scheme, is a hard-won understanding that our natural inclinations have wise purposes demanding respect even if not yet fully plumbed. Such an understanding is only confirmed when the technical or social sciences uncover new functions of what man does by mere inclination. In fact, that is one of the most important roles for those sciences.

The "higher education" deplored by Ratner tends less toward respecting nature than manipulating it. It burdens its students with the stultifying task of mastering nature without first obeying its laws. It is the education that has been offered at most American universities since roughly the turn of the century when they adopted the German model with its emphasis on

3 "The Natural Institution of the Family Challenged", *Journal of the North American Montessori Teacher's Association*, 19,2,p.122.
Dr. Ratner is quoting from Fragment 327 of Pascal's *Pensees* in the Every man's translation by W.F. Trotter. It reads in part:
"...The sciences have two extremes which meet. The first is the pure Natural ignorance in which all men find themselves at birth. The other Extreme is that reached by great intellects, who, having run through all that men can know, find they know nothing, and come back again to that same ignorance from which they set out; but this is a learned ignorance which is conscious of itself. Those between the two, who have departed from natural ignorance and not been able to reach the other, have some smatter of this vain knowledge, and pretend to be wise. These trouble the world and are bad judges of everything."

the physical and social sciences, and on research. The German university and its American counterpart take their character from the rationalist current of the Enlightenment, hence ignore the kinds of knowledge stemming from affinity (such as the "connatural knowledge" of Thomas Aquinas) or from instinct or emotion (such as the "empathy" of Edith Stein and other phenomenologists).[4] More traditional education, based largely on this the Aristotelian tradition, respects instinct and emotion, and holds that they have much to teach us.

Efforts to restore the broader and deeper education traditionally called "liberal," which predominated in this country until late in the last century, have in isolated instances been brilliantly successful, but Ratner held that on the widespread re-establishment of such education hangs the restoration of medicine, of the ethos, independence, and esteem once characteristic of the profession.

Even the very effectiveness of medicine, paradoxical as it may seem in this day of dazzling technology, also depends on the restoration of liberal education and the philosophy it fosters. The principal reason that such sound philosophy is vital to the effectiveness of medicine is that it grasps the role of teleology—that is, intrinsic purpose—in nature, thereby acknowledging the body itself as the prime healer. Hence technology, whose limitations are revealed with its every advance, that is every time it leaves its previous achievements behind, takes second place.

In conversations on the respective roles of nature and technology, Dr.

---

4   Probably the most frequently cited passage from Aquinas on connatural knowledge is from the *Summa theologiae* II-II, 45.2:

> "...Right judgment...can occur in two ways: one, by the perfect use of reason; the other, because of a certain connaturality with those things about which one has to judge. Just as he who has dedicated himself to moral science judges rightly by rational enquiry those things pertaining to chastity, so but through a certain connaturality to those things, does the man with the habit of chastity judge rightly about them."

To grasp St. Thomas's point, we must bear in mind that habit, for him, is a kind of second nature." The least that can be said here is that the "second nature" of the virtue of chastity steadies a man's judgment about the rightness or wrongness of genital behavior. St. Thomas is supplying a reason for the Aristotelean dictum that if you want to know the right thing to do, consult the just man.

For knowledge through empathy, see Edith Stein, *On the Problem of Empathy*, transl. Waltraut Stein, (The Hague: Martinus Nijhoff, 1964) ch. IV; also translator's introduction, esp. pp. XVII and XVIII. For a history of the concept in psychology and philosophy, see Nancy Eisenberg and Janet Strayer, eds., *Empathy and Its Development* (Cambridge: Cambridge University Press, 1987), ch, 2.

Ratner illustrated how the Hippocratic philosophy resists the technological imperative.

> **Disease can overwhelm nature. A basic principle of the Art of medicine is to do for nature what nature would do for itself if it could. But a tendency of physicians is to intervene before intervention is necessary.**

Here he cited obstetrics, which he said "tends to be largely interventionist, because man is impatient, and nature seems to be too slow." He cautioned:

> **But interventionist medicine can end up substituting for nature, as far example in Caesarians. If you know how to do a Caesarian, and do it well, you enjoy doing it, so there's an advantage to home delivery. An episiotomy is rarely necessary, but you're tempted to say "Why wait?" You must give nature a chance.**

If you put interventionism to one side, he added, you end up with natural Childbirth.

> **It took a long time to realize that the tonsils are an important part of the lymphatic system, protecting against disease such as bulbar polio. Often we fail to understand the function of a part of the body until we lose that part, as for example when we found that the loss of the thyroid led to myxedema.**

In that, said Ratner, the body is like a great work of art:

> **Mozart is a good example. It's difficult to know what makes art great because all the parts work together. Imperfect art gives you insights into great art.**

Here he cited Beethoven and Brahms as offering insights, by the imperfections of their art, into the perfect art of Mozart. (One need not concur with the examples to grasp the principle.)

Still on the theme of the body as its own healer, he asked why a patient goes to a doctor. His answer: "A distressing symptom."

The prevailing philosophy is that a doctor has a medication for every symptom. If its fever, we start with the notion of fighting it, and forget that fever is a curative factor of nature. We don't think of symptoms as curative, but we should bear in mind that they are.

When the patient leaves the doctor's office with only the advice to wait patiently and get back to him if the symptoms don't disappear, he may think the doctor has done nothing for him. On the other hand:

If he leaves with a piece of paper, he's more likely to feel satisfied. Writing a prescription is the fastest way of getting a patient out of your office. The hardest thing in medicine is to do nothing.

Isn't there a very important role for medicines, and for Surgery?

No question. To help nature you need techniques. You must be competent . This is the premise. As a non-surgeon, you must know what surgery might be indicated. I need a surgeon who'll go my way in terms of my clinical judgment.

(This is in accord with the Hippocratic notion of surgery as a secondary art, dependent on the physician.)

But "this day of synthetic drugs," he said, brings its own problems.

The body isn't constituted to handle them to detoxify itself of them. They baffle the liver.[5]

---

5   A study published April 15, 1989 by the *Journal of the American Medical Association* reported that more than 100,000 patients a year die in U.S. hospitals form drug reactions. That would make adverse reaction to medication a leading cause of death in America.

An author of the report, Dr. Bruce Pomeranz, said: "We want to increase awareness that drugs have a toxic component." He hold *The New York Times* of April 15 that drug reaction was underreported as a cause of death because it is rarely reported on the death certificate, which might list stomach hemorrhage as the cause of death without mentioning that the hemorrhage was caused by a drug. He estimated that there were from 76,000 to 137,000 deaths from medication a year,

He recalled that one of his first practical lessons as a young physician was to remove all medication from a patient who was taking five or six different kinds of pill. He found, for example, that some prescriptions were written to counter the unwanted effects of an earlier prescription, as when an insomniac patient on a sedative is given a stimulant to counteract the resulting dopeyness.

But some prescriptions do damage by their very nature.

The best example is drugs messing up a woman's hormonal system. When the Pill came out, I told Chris Knott *(the late Msgr. John C. Knott, director of the Family Life Office of the United States Catholic Conference)* that the trouble with it was giving a powerful drug to healthy women.

This, he pointed out, is diametrically opposed to the Hippocratic philosophy of medicine. (He observed parenthetically that widespread use of the birth control pill has meant higher concentrations of female hormones in the water supply.)

To ignore the structure and functions of the human body, he held, is to opt for second best at best. As a lifelong advocate of breast-feeding, he went the length of holding that no reform would accomplish more for the future of the nation than the restoration of breast-feeding. (It might, for example, be argued that the trust in others implanted in a child from his earliest days is an effective antidote to the Hobbesian notion of society, which requires a Leviathan-like state to protect men from one another.)

---

while the number of deaths attributed to that cause on death certificates in 1994 was 156.

Dr. Pomeranz, a professor of neuroscience, and his colleagues at the University of Toronto combined the results of 39 smaller studies in a technique called meta-analysis, which gives researchers the possibility of drawing statistically significant conclusions. The method has its critics, and the authors noted that the results of their study should be taken viewed with caution.

This was echoed by an editorial in the *Journal* by Dr. David Bates, an associate professor of medicine at Harvard. According to the Times, Dr. Bates speculated that the death rate reported in Dr. Pomeranz's study might be exaggerated because the study focused on large teaching hospitals with the sickest patients. Patients in intensive care, he noted , might receive 20 to 40 drugs. He said that drugs probably save millions of lives yearly. Drs. Bates and Pomeranz agreed that benefits from drugs far exceed risks in the great majority of cases.

In 1957 he helped found the La Leche League for the promotion of breast-feeding, and he was a consultant for the remaining 40 years of his life.

He was fond of pointing out that there seems to be no end to the nutrition found in mother's milk, including hormones regulating the proper growth of the child. Moreover breast-feeding fortifies the bond between mother and child.

> **For example, the newborn baby's focal length is the distance from his eyes to the mother's face when nursing. The peripheral vision is blocked out... The baby, like the horse on the road, has blinders, to speak. Nature does this for the baby so that the baby can concentrate on the mother—its rock of refuge from whom the newborn learns trust and fidelity, which will serve him in good stead in future human relations.**[6]

Ratner goes further, holding that to ignore the structure and functions of the human body may be inviting disaster.

> **Any fool should know that the vagina is the organ to receive the inseminating organ, and therefore is the repository of the semen. Apart from morals, the physician as biologist should recognize that to put the penis in the anus, and deposit semen in the rectum, is to court medical difficulties.**

> **You must realize that everything nature does is exquisite in terms of subtleties, complexities. Semen, which for the most part has held the interest of gynecologists only with respect to the sperm and sterility, is 82 percent plasma. We should realize that the plasma given by nature has multiple functions. I'll mention only one.**

> **The sperm and the embryo are foreign bodies in the woman, and have to be protected against the woman's immune system, which builds up antibodies against the sperm and the embryo. We've known from clinical experience, and in more recent years through chemical studies, that when a woman is pregnant she's more susceptible to lots of diseases because the semen suppresses in part the immune system of her body.**

---

6   *The Natural Institution of the Family Challenged,* Journal of the North American Montessori Teachers' Association., p. 143.

What is this substance in the semen that suppresses the immune system ? The plasma of semen has the highest concentration of prostaglandins in the human body. You must bear in mind that every secretion is a prescription of nature, and like a doctor's prescription has reasons for every ingredient.

Beyond that, there's an organ. The vagina is constructed to accommodate this process (of immunosupression), so that the immune suppressant is modes and modulated. The vaginal wall is thicker than the membrane of the anus. The vaginal membrane is composed of squamous cells, overlapping like singles on a roof. That manages to produce a mild depressant of the immune system. You know as a biologist the anus is essentially an outlet, and its thinner membrane is very absorbent since the rectum extracts various things from the waste products. The vagina is essentially an inlet, and absorbs plasma slowly.

Moral theologians of times past may have been wiser than they knew when they wrote of the *vas indebitum,* the "undue vessel."

Dr. Ratner, remarking that the most prevalent way of contracting AIDS is via the anus, asserted that anal intercourse is not exclusive to homosexual acts but probably accounts for ten or twenty percent of heterosexual intercourse in this country, and higher percentage abroad.

There are "two major scandals" in what is called AIDS education, he said: first in not making it abundantly clear that the prime way of spreading the AIDS virus is anal intercourse, and then, second is assuming that all heterosexual intercourse is vaginal.

The Hippocratic physician, Ratner held, counsels his patients not only to respect nature but to strengthen it as well:

The Hippocratic order of treatment began with a Regimen. You got a good sleep, ate well, relaxed after work, and exercised.

Than came medicine, and finally surgery. Today the tendency is to reverse the order: the surgeon, then the doctor, then the regimen. Just recently I read that if you follow a good regimen, you can dispense with most drugs for high blood-pressure.

In this context the title given a physician is significant, according to Ratner:

Doctor means teacher. The doctor should educate his patients in conservative ways to maintain health. This is where regimen is the best prescription: rest, eat properly, and exercise.

But fidelity to the name of doctor is not, in Ratner's view, characteristic of medicine today:

This is an age of iatrogenic medicine, of diseases caused by medical treatment. It's one of the worst periods in history for medicine. A new book by a heart specialist, *(Dryden)* Morse, holds that medications for heart disease are responsible for 50,000 deaths yearly in this country.

Dr. Ratner's concern about the technological imperative can be seen in the Ratnerian paradox: "Every advance is a setback…." Pause. Then, mischievously, "…unless you're a Hippocratic physician."

Ratner himself was a protagonist in what is probably the foremost example of a medical advance that proved a setback, the introduction of the Salk Vaccine against poliomyelitis. Dr. Eugene Diamond writes:

On April 12, 1955, there was a nationwide telecast of the Results of the 1954 field trials of the Salk Vaccine. It was called "The Medical Story of the Century" and, in terms of the huge promotion and publicity given to the announcement, that description of the event was not hyperbole.

Herbert Ratner was, at the time, Director of Public Health in Oak Park, Illinois, and the Editor of the *Bulletin Of the American Association of Public Health Physicians.* His questioning of the methodology and the soundness of the

science which produced the data is one of the great stories of clinical integrity of the last 50 years.

His position, taken in the face of overwhelming opposition, was soon vindicated by the occurrence of vaccine-induced cases of poliomyelitis. It is a dramatic untold story which is not yet fully played out as scientists continue to question the long-term significance of the contamination of the Salk Vaccine with Simian Virus 40.[7]

Medicine became a profession, Ratner never tired of recalling, precisely because its members professed an oath. Moreover medicine was the first calling to require an oath of its members, and hence was the first profession. The other profession that followed – the learned profession of law and divinity, and the military—all became professions because they too took oaths. Not surprisingly, these oaths are modeled on the Hippocratic Oath of the Physician.

Any professional oath, Ratner maintained, is a bulwark against "the vagaries of society." That is why, when such "vagaries" infect a profession, the tendency is to "update" the oath or dismiss it as a quaint relic of a less enlightened age.

Nor was Ratner at a loss for historical examples. In 1972, he published a informal protest made by Dutch physicians during the Nazi occupation of the Netherlands against a supervising body that the German authorities were about to impose on the Dutch medical profession. It read in part:

We know that you represent a very special philosophy of life. Our knowledge of the German "physicians' ordinance" concerning the task of the physician in which the care for race and nation takes precedence over that of the individual, makes it only too clear to what extent the national-socialistic (nazi) conception of medical profession differs from ours.

Although we do not deny that the care of the community and the participation in social hygiene measures constitute part of the task of the physician, we can recognize this duty only insofar as it proceeds from and is not in conflict with the first and holiest precept of the physician, namely the respect

---

7   Editor's Note in *Nature, the Physician, and the Family* (Rockford, Illinois: TAN Books, 1990), the collected works of Herbert Ratner.

for life and for the physical well-being of the individual who entrusts himself to his care....

Knowing ourselves bound by the oath or solemn vow of acceptance of our task as physicians, we consider it our duty to inform you that we shall remain faithful to the high standards which have been the foundation of our profession since time immemorial....[8]

Dr. Ratner observed:

This protest underscores the *raison d'ete* of the document, which today is undergoing attack from brave new crops of medical students, professors of obstetrics turned sociologists, social ethicist reformers, population engineers, less than thoughtful segments of the women's liberation movement, crusading lawyer-simplifiers of criminal codes, and abortionists and 'mercy' killers...

As sensitivities atrophy, and the concept of natural holiness weakens, as the scorn of God and religion intensifies, we should once again ask ourselves, "Who are the victors of World War II?"[9]

Naturally the question arises whether medicine even remains a profession when the oath becomes little more than a memory, either through institutionalized disregard of its provisions or by dispensing with it altogether. Equivalent to this latter course is the substitution of other "declarations" at the graduation ceremonies of medical schools.

A "declaration" is not an oath, nor is a solemn pledge or a promise. In none of these does the promisor, the pledger, or the declarer swear by some higher power, such as the gods of Greece or the God of Abraham, Isaac, and Jacob. He does not appeal to what he holds most sacred to witness his resolve to keep his word. Neither does he, according to the timeless formula, call down upon himself a blessing if faithful to what he has sworn, and a curse if unfaithful.

8   "Dutch Physicians' Protest Against Nazi Regulations," *Child & Family*, Vol. 11, No. 2, 1972. The review, edited by Dr. Ratner, said the statement was "reprinted from *Repression and Resistance – The Netherlands in Time of War*, Vol. II, p.352," and that the translator was Conrad W. Baars, M.D.

9   Ibid.

Moreover the contents of the various substitutes for the Hippocratic Oath incorporate dilutions of distortions to one degree or another. The so-called Declaration of Geneva, adopted in 1948 by the General Assembly of the World Medical Association in Geneva, was meant to replace the Hippocratic Oath on entry into the medical profession. Its grandiloquent phrases—"consecrate my life to the service of humanity," and "maintain by all the means in my power the honor and the noble traditions of the medical profession"—are but vague substitutes for the hard specifics of the Hippocratic Oath. They can scarcely erect the same moral defenses around the medical profession. Nor has the Geneva Declaration stood fast against agitation to relax its moral demands.

Dr. Ratner recalled that although the Declaration of Geneva was designed to reinvigorate the medical profession after the disclosures of the Nuremberg trials, pro-abortion and pro-euthanasia forces were already active during its drafting.

I remember reading in the foreign correspondence of the AMA that originally there was no reference to killing. They were going to get rid of the prohibition. It was the Latin American countries that complained.

As published in 1948, the Geneva Declaration stipulates: "I will maintain the utmost respect for human life, from the time of conception, even under threat." This adds the ethical element of resistance to threat, and the scientific understanding that human life begin at conception, to the Hippocratic requirement that the physician swear: "I will give no deadly medicine to anyone if asked, nor suggest any such counsel; and in like manner I will not give a woman a pessary to produce an abortion." On the other hand the Oath, as can be seen, is more specific in excluding complicity in abortion and suicide.

But agitators have been at work since 1948. Subsequent version of the Geneva Declaration reveal that, as an artifact of the times rather than a monument of antiquity, it has not been proof against ideology. It has been amended in 1968, 1983, and 1994. The latest version would be labeled in the vocabulary of our times as politically correct. It incorporates the ideologically-battered science promoted by advocates of abortion: instead of pledging to "maintain the utmost respect for human life from the time of conception," it now refers to "human life from its beginning" (whenever or whatever that may be, or may prove to be with the next shift in ideology). Moreover "gender" and "sexual orientation" (meaning sexual disorientation) have worked their way among the considerations that the physician may not allow "to intervene between my duty and my patient."

The vicissitudes of the Geneva Declaration since its approval half a century ago support the wisdom of leaving well enough alone. Little wonder that the gods of Greece remained at the head of the Hippocratic Oath throughout the most Christian ages.

A modified oath, taken in recent years by medical students at graduation (if indeed any oath is taken), appears to subsume the Hippocratic Oath's prohibition of euthanasia and abortion under an undertaking to "perform no operation, for a criminal purpose, even if solicited, far less suggest it."[10] This of course leaves the purely healing and health-preserving character of the medical profession at the mercy of civil law, for if abortion or euthanasia is legal, then the physician can plead that he is bound by no oath against it. Civil authorities can make the same argument should they demand that physicians commit legally-sanctioned crimes forbidden by the Hippocratic Oath but not by a modified oath.

Even weaker in this regard are the American Medical Association's "Principles of Medical Ethics," which merely demand that a physician "respect the law" and "the rights of patients, of colleagues, and of other health professionals." The AMA's "Principles of Medical Ethics make another bow to whatever the civil law may stipulate, possibly at the expense of medical ethics or even of natural justice, in requiring that the physician "safeguard patient confidences within the constraints of the law." The Oath on the other hand burdens the physician with a fully moral obligation to keep secret "whatever in connection with my professional practice or not in connection with it" that "ought not to be spoken abroad." Civil law, far from getting pride of place, does not even enter in.

Where the Geneva Declaration has the physician undertake to "practice my profession with conscience and dignity," the Hippocratic Oath has him swear not only to practice his art "with purity and holiness" but also to pass his life in that same purity and that same holiness. The Oath seems more realistic in the sense that one can hardly be a pillar of ethics in the clinic and a moral mess at home. Moreover purity and holiness of life are hardly compatible with the abortion that the American Medical Association has not only tolerated, not only promoted, but even attempted to force upon medical schools and their students.

A somewhat mysterious document called the Prayer—or sometimes

---

10   Reproduced in *Healthline* March 1995.,

the Oath—of Maimonides is if anything even more elevated spiritually than the Hippocratic Oath.[11] But it is in no way an oath, for it does not call upon God to witness the truth of a pledge. Rather it begs Him for light and for strength of body and soul, hence must be considered a prayer. About twice the length of the Hippocratic Oath, it can be described as a detailed petition for the virtues required of a physician.

Two such virtues received explicit recognition in the Hippocratic Oath: absolute discretion about private matters learned in the practice of the profession, and sexual purity. In the Oath the physician swears to shun "the seduction of females or males," whether free or slave. Whereas one modern version of the Oath tendered new physicians demands that they abstain "from the tempting of others to vice," the AMA Principles of Medical Ethics breathe not a word about sexual misbehavior, which as Ratner often pointed out is an occupational hazard for physicians.

Given the role of the Hippocratic Oath in maintaining the character of medicine as a healing profession, not killing profession, it's no surprise that the U. S. Supreme Court, in attempting to justify medically-induced abortion, attacked the Oath. It was not a frontal assault; the opinion fairly glowed with veneration for Hippocrates, but it attempted to cut the historical ground out from under the Oath.

The Court did this by citing an historian of medicine, Ludwig Edelstein, who argued that the Oath incorporated the ethical precepts of a particular philosophical school, the Pythagoreans, and moreover at a particular time, the fourth century B.C.

Said the Court:

> **Dr. Edelstein then concludes that the Oath originated in a group representing only a small segment of Greek opinion and that it certainly was not accepted by all ancient physicians.... But with the end of antiquity a decided change took place. Resistance against suicide and against abortion became common. The Oath came to be popular. The emerging teachings of Christianity were in agreement with the Pythagorean ethic. The Oath "became the nucleus of all medical ethics" and "was applauded as the embodiment of truth." Thus, suggests Dr. Edelstein, it is "a Pythagorean manifest and not the expression of an absolute Standard of medical conduct."**

---

11   As well as being a physician, Moses Maimonides (1135-1204) was a philosopher and theologian highly regarded by Christian theologians of the Middle Ages. St. Thomas quotes him often, under the name of Rabbi Moses.

This, it seems to us, is a satisfactory and acceptable explanation of the Hippocratic Oath's apparent rigidity.[12]

In this way, the abortionist Court was able to wave aside two millennia of medical tradition and, thus unimpeded, launch its assault on the medical profession.

For irony, it would be hard to beat the case of Ludwig Edelstein. He had a foresight to flee Nazi Germany, yet it is an essay of his that has given scholarly color to the campaign against the very tradition that surely, had it been maintained, would have saved many of his fellow Jews. The reason seems to be that he was unaware, like the rest of the world, of the depth of evil then holding sway in Germany. He published his study in 1943, before the depth of the betrayal of German medicine had been made clear.

Moreover, according to the editors of the posthumous collection of Dr. Edelstein's studies on ancient medicine in which the essay was eventually republished, until his death he remained undecided about it. If that last sentence is not clear, neither were the editors, Owsei and C. Lilian Temkin, in explaining Edelstein's state of mind. Their carefully worded introduction leaves the reader in doubt about the focus of Edelstein's indecision: was it *where* to include the essay on the Oath in the book, or *whether* to include it?

They write:

The present volume contains those essays available after his death which Edelstein himself had considered for inclusion. It presents them in the four sections under which he had subsumed them.[13]

They add in a footnote: "With the exception of *The Hippocratic Oath*, on which he had not reached a decision."

In either case—that is, *where* or *whether* Edelstein wanted the essay republished—the inclusion of "The Hippocratic Oath" in *Ancient Medicine* was to lift this momentous essay from the obscurity of a supplement to the *Bulletin of the History of Medicine*. With or without his approval, Edelstein's "The Hippocratic Oath" went before a broader public in 1967, two years

12   *Roe v. Wade*, 410U.S. 130, 93 S.Ct. 705 (1973), at 132.

13   Edelstein, L., *Ancient Medicine*, eds. Owsei Temkin and C. Lillian Temkin, transl. C. Lilian Temkin (Baltimore: John Hopkins Press, 1967), p. xii, Editors' Introduction.

after he died. The editors gave it pride of place: It is the opening essay of the book.

On the more likely reading that Edelstein never authorized the republication of his study, we can wonder why he hesitated. We can even wonder whether he did not eventually determine to withhold the work. Why might he do either? Or dread of what uses it might be put to?[14]

In the event, the republished essay not only was cited by the Supreme Court in striking down virtually all laws prohibiting or regulating abortion but was earlier exploited by Laurence Lader in his successful agitation for legal abortion in this country, and was appealed to in France during the equally successful campaign to legalize abortion there.

It is certain that Edelstein would have been appalled by the distortion of his study into a weapon in the worldwide campaign for abortion. He venerated the Oath. We find him in 1956 declaring himself "second to none in my appreciation of this document."[15] Clearly he recognized that whatever the provenance or original purpose or date of the document—the three points he attempted to establish in his study—none of these, whatever they might be, could detract from the decisive role the Hippocratic Oath has played in forging the character of Western medicine, hence of Western civilization. Nor could they, whatever they might be, dilute, devalue, or destroy the ethical principles of the Oath, which became, in Edelstein's works, "the nucleus of all medical ethics."[16] He writes:

> **In all countries, in all epochs in which monotheism, in its purely religious or in its more secularized form, was the accepted creed, the Hippocratic Oath was applauded as the embodiment of truth. Not only Jews and Christians, but the Arabs..., scientists of the Enlightenment, and scholars of the nineteenth century embraced the ideals of the Oath.**[17]

---

14   Prophetically, one might think, Edelstein held that two stipulations of the Oath "seem to point to the basic beliefs underlying the whole program," namely renunciation of complicity in suicide and in abortion" (op. cit., p.8). Hence he held that they could "provide a clue for historical identification of the views embodied in the Oath of Hippocrates," and based his study and his conclusions on that clue.

15   Op. cit., p. 327, in "The Professional Ethics of the Greek Physician." This lecture was first published in the *Bulletin of the History of Medicine,* 1956, Vol. 30, pp. 391-419.

16   Op. cit., p. 63, in "the Hippocratic Oath."

17   Ibid.

This is not the place to examine Dr. Edelstein's celebrated study in any detail, but a few more observations may help keep it in perspective.

Edelstein himself, deservedly or not early had a not altogether enviable reputation for "constant deviation from accepted views' and for presenting his arguments 'as cogent demonstrations with inescapable results."[18]

On a more substantive matter, he betrays a basic if only too common misunderstanding of the nature of medicine, characterizes medicine as "a craft," "the physician as "a craftsman."[19] This is no translator's error: not only did Edelstein scrutinize and emend all English translations of his work, but he actually delved into Aristotle's treatment of crafts as indicative of the esteem for medicine in Aristotle's time, and held that the Pythagorean and Stoic, and the later Hellenistic philosophies, confirmed such esteem by upholding the dignity of the craftsman's work.[20]

Now a significant characteristic of the Hippocratic Oath is to call medicine "the Art." This term is used for medicine throughout the writings of the Hippocratic school, including the Oath itself. To call medicine an art may not seem very helpful since the word has a multiplicity of meanings; unless the meaning of art is historically and contextually clarified, to speak of medicine as an art can and usually does cause confusion.

As etymological approach to the concept of medicine-as-art can only confuse us. First, *art* is the root of *artisan,* and it was Edelstein's apparent error to call the physician a craftsman, that is an artisan. Moreover the Greek work for art, *techne,* gave us our word *technology.* Yet every Hippocratic physician is aware that if his profession becomes mere technology, he might as well hand it over to diagnostic devices and computers.[21]

Moderns who seek the significance of medicine-as-art must look less to linguistics than to Greek philosophy. In the mind of Aristotle, art and

18   Editors; introduction to *Ancient Medicine,* p. ix.

19   *Ancient Medicine,* passim.

20   Op. cit., pp. 327-328, in The Professional Ethics of the Greek Physician." For Edelstein's attention to translations, see editors' introduction, p. xiii.

21   An article in the *New York Times,* Dec. 16, 1997, "New Way of Doctoring: By the Book," discusses attempts to harness the medical research available on the internet, and to base treatment on it. It is termed "evidence-based medicine." The writer, Abigail Zuger, quotes a comment by Dr. Sandra J. Tanenbaum of Ohio State College of Medicine that "no one thing works for everyone all the time," adding that that's where the art of Medicine comes in.

To this Dr. David Sackett, director of he Centre for Evidence-Based Medicine in Oxford, England, responded, "art kills." He added:

"It was the art that gave us purging, puking, leeches, the gastric freeze, all that sort of stuff....There's a science to the art of Medicine."

science are, both of them, kinds of knowledge: an art is knowledge for the sake of producing something, while a science is knowledge for its own sake. Science finds sits fulfillment in knowledge gained, art in a product produced.

Ratner explains the distinction in terms characteristically homely, clear, and memorable:

> **Man is a wondering animal. Unlike other animals he cannot live in the world without wanting to explain it. Man is also a making animal. Unlike other animals he cannot live in the world without wanting to improve it. As a wondering animal he seeks the reason behind the fact. His goal is truth. As a making animal he seeks the means to accomplish the end; His goal is the good.**
>
> **Both activities are functions of his intellect. Traditionally, these different operations of the mind are distinguished as the work of the theoretical or speculative intellect and the work of the practical activity, when perfected, characterizes man as a scientist; the latter, as an artist.[22]**

In the case of medicine, the artist finds his fulfillment in producing health, that is in sustaining it or restoring it. In the case of law, the fulfillment is to produce justice, that is, to uphold or restore it. Neither justice nor health, however, can be called an artifact, which is what is produced by the artisan, the craftsman working on inert matter.

If art is simply the right way of making something, and if a singe word *(techne)* was used by Greeks both for a craft and for a fine art, how then explain the transcendental leap form the homely art of the artisan to the ineffable art of a Mozart, a Michelangelo, a Shakespeare? This obviously is a significant question in the attempt to understand what the Hippocratic tradition means in calling medicine "the Art."

To untangle this question we might first clarify how artists in the more rudimentary sense of those who produce something can differ among themselves. Here Aristotle, significantly at the outset of his twelve books of metaphysics, provides us with a hierarchy of distinctions:

---

22 "The Oath—V. Why?" *Child & Family,* Vol. 10, No.4, 1971, p. 290. This is the fifth in a series of six articles by Dr. Ratner on the Hippocratic Oath.

...the man of experience *(empeiros)* appears wiser than those who just have some power of sensation or other, the artist *(technites)* than men of experience, the master builder *(architekton)* than the handicraftsman *(cheirotechnes)*, and the theoretical sciences *(theoretikai...epistemai)* than the productive *(poietika)*.[23]

Aristotle had already met the objection that a man of experience may prove more capable of effective action than the theoretician. There, not surprisingly, he used medicine as his example. He begins:

...we see men of experience succeeding more than those who have theory without experience. The reason for this is that experience is knowledge of particulars, but art of universals; and actions and the effects produced are all concerned with the particular.[24]

Aristotle then offers his well-known aphorism:

For it is not man that the physician cures, except incidentally, but Callias or Socrates or some other like-named person, who is incidentally a man as well. So if a man has theory without experience, and knows the universal *but does not know the particular contained in it,* he will often fail in his treatment, for it is the particular that must be treated.[25]

Where does this leave the artist who has a grasp of principles?

Aristotle observes:

Nevertheless we consider that knowledge and proficiency belong to art rather than to experience, and we assume that artists are wiser than men of mere experience...: and this is because the former know the cause, whereas the latter do not. For men of experience know the fact, but not the wherefore; but artists know the wherefore and the cause.[26]

23   *I Metaphysics* I, I (981b29-982al).
24   Op. cit., (1981a14—18).
25   Op. cit., (19-24).
26   Op. cit., (24-30).

With such common objections overcome, Aristotle can then claim, as he did in the passage quoted previously, not just the superiority of experience over animal instinct or sensation, but the superiority of theoretical knowledge over experience.

In that same passage he moves on to two distinct kinds of worker, the master-builder *(architekton)* and the artisan, whose Greek name *cheirtochnes* means literally "hand-artist" and might be rendered "handicraftsman." He has mentioned them earlier, and has already supported his next claim, that the master-builder is wiser than the handicraftsman, on grounds that master-builders "know the reasons for the tings that are done, but we think that the handicraftsmen, like inanimate objects, do things but without knowing what they are doing..., through habit."[27]

If a knowledge of the reasons for doing things sets the master-builder apart from the handicraftsman, is that same knowledge what sets the sculptor apart from his stonecarvers, or the physician apart from the aides and technicians he may employ? In part, yes, for physician and sculptor alike understand causes that their technically skilled helpers, however intelligent and productive, may not. But the specific difference between the true artist and the artisan, as indeed between the true artist and the master-builder, has to be sought elsewhere. It is found in the material, so to seek, that the true artist works on: human nature itself.

Thus the clearest exemplar of the true artist is the physician. He works on the human being, in cooperation with that purposeful inner activity—or entelechy, to use Aristotelian term in its more modern, vitalistic sense—which is proper to all living things.

St. Thomas, distinguishing between arts that work upon inert matter, such as wood and stone for the art of building, and arts that work upon "an active principle tending to produce the effect of the art," takes medicine for his example of the latter:

Such is the medical art, since in the sick body there is an active principle conducive to health. Hence the effect of art of the first kind (working on inert matter) is never produced by nature but is always the result of the art; every house is an artifact. But the effect of the art of the second kind is the result both of art and of nature without art; for many are cured by the action of nature without the art of medicine.

---

27   Op. cit., (981b2-5).

Now in those things which can be done both by art and by nature, art imitates nature.[28]

To fill out the picture a word must be said about other arts such as that of the jurist and those of the composer, poet, painter and sculptor. The last two are manifestly imitative of nature. Since Aristotle's *Poetics* at least, the notion of the art as the imitation of nature has held pride of place, but it has been applied chiefly if not exclusively to the esthetic arts.[29] The *Poetics*, a fragmentary work of which we possess perhaps half, has aided and abetted this narrow view by dealing less with the analysis of principles than with their application to poetry and music, and to the artistic conventions of the author's day. Yet implicit throughout the book, and explicit often enough, is the principle that the artist of every kind, through what he produces in imitation of human life, aims at affecting human nature.

By their nature, the esthetic arts first affect the emotions, but the classic view, embodied in the civic theater and civic architecture of Athens, and in the cathedrals and morality plays of the Middle Ages, has been that such arts answer their finest calling when they bring the right emotions to the aid of principle, thus creating conviction. Or perhaps when the physician uses them as part of his therapeutic regimen.

We can see that what constitutes the specific difference between an art in the more inclusive and homely sense and an art in the more exclusive and higher sense is twofold: the artist's knowledge of the beauty and that affects our emotions, and his ability to bring that beauty into being. When a beautifully designed building is directed at our senses, and through them elevates our spirit much as does music or poetry, architecture moves beyond the task of an artisan or even a master-builder to the achievement of an artist. In other words, the transcendental (or "quantum") leap to pure

28   *Summa contra gentiles*, II 75, 15.

29   *Poetics*, iii, 4, begins as follows:
> "It is clear that the general origin of poetry was due to two causes, each of them part of human nature. Imitation is natural to man from childhood, one of his advantages over the lower animals being this, that he is the most imitative creature in the world, and learns at first by imitation. And it is also natural for all to delight in works of imitation…. The explanation is to be found in a further fact: to be learning something is the greatest of pleasures not only to the philosopher but also to the rest of mankind, however small their capacity for it…" (1448b1-5).

(I have followed the translation of Ingraham Bywater because its rendering of *mineomai* and its cognates in terms of *imitation* rather than *representation* not only fits the text better but more fully substantiates our point.)

art is made when the worker knowingly brings his skills to bear on human nature, stimulating and harnessing, so to speak, its powers.

Here we can discern that the concept of art is as important for a right understanding of law as it is of medicine. In the art of the jurist the mind puts our natural thirst for justice, and out rational grasp of the intrinsically right thing, to work in the affairs of men to set them right, thus safeguarding or restoring the health of society. Jurisprudence works with nature in what can be considered its highest activity, namely the production of virtue.

This stands athwart the currently dominant philosophy of law, called Legal Positivism (or sometimes Historicism, a quite similar thing), which conceives law as an artifact produced by and out of the arbitrary will of the lawmaker, or as another variant would have it, of the judge. The Roman jurists, on the contrary, spoke of law as turning the establishment of the intrinsically right thing into an art—*jus redigere in artem*—much as we can say Hippocratic medicine turns the preservation and restoration of health into an art.

This classic notion of art, needless to say, has just about evaporated from the minds of us moderns. Nor is our understanding of the tradition that law and medicine are arts given much help when we learn that the liberal arts, the study of which is according to Ratner the best preparation for the study of medicine, are really sciences. The are called arts by analogy.

Sometimes the analogy is construed as illustrating that the liberal arts produce educated men, or knowledge that can be considered useful. St. Thomas proposes a closer parallel: The seven liberal arts of grammar, logic, rhetoric, arithmetic, geometry, music, and astronomy are called arts because "they not only have knowledge but a certain product." Grammar is said to produce a properly constructed sentence, logic correct reasoning, rhetoric a speech, and so forth.[30]

In any case, what we get is a mish-mash: medicine, nowadays called a science, is in the classical tradition an art, while the liberal arts, traditionally the best preparation for medical studies, are sciences in the classical sense.

An essay called simply "The Art" ("Peri Technes") is one of the better-

---

30   In *Boetii de Trinitate* Vol. 1, ad 3.

For much the same argument see *Summa theologiae* I-II, 57, 3, ad 3. There St. Thomas also holds that they are called "liberal" to distinguish them from "those Arts which are ordered to works carried out by the body, which are in a certain sense 'servile' insofar as the body is subject to the soul as a servant, and man is free (*liber*) because of his soul."

known writings in the Hippocratic corpus. For the Hippocratic physician, medicine is the art par excellence. Yet so firmly locked n the modern psyche is a notion of art as a knack perfected by practice, or as a preternatural gift given a Mozart or a Michelangelo, that translators of the essay—not a work of Hippocrates, by the way—actually changed title and text alike to conform with the notion that medicine is, in their term, "an exact science." Moreover they twist and turn to avoid the wordplay that opens the essay: "Some there are who have made an art of vilifying the arts...." The translators wrestle this into banality: "There are men who have made a business of abusing the sciences."[31]

Misreading of the nature of medicine are practically the rule. In the past two centuries and more, since the "scientific" side of medicine revealed its wonders and began its triumphal march, medicine has been progressively abandoning its Hippocratic self-understanding. That means, chiefly, retreat from *nature* in its manifold functions: first, as the prime healer to be aided by the art of the physician; then as the standard of normality, to be aimed at by the physician in his art; and last though by no means least as the standard of ethics, to be defended by him as if the very life of medicine depended on it. And so it does, for if medicine is no longer a moral art, it is no longer a living profession.

---

31   Chadwick, John, and W.N. Mann, *The Medical Works of Hippocrates* (Oxford: Blackwell, 1950), p. 81.

CHAPTER 6

A FUTURE FOR MEDICINE?

By

Nigel Cameron, PhD

Paternalism and Pluralism

More than one recent writer has drawn attention to the fact that contemporary discussions of medical ethics are largely taken up with questions of procedure. Rather than address the substantive ethical issues which are focused by technical developments and general ethical flux, physicians and ethicists alike respond by concentrating on the way in which decisions are made. The explanation is plain. We live in a society in which agreement about what it is right to do is increasingly hard to find. It is easier to agree on the procedures which will allow individuals to make their own free choices. With the ebbing of the western ethical consensus it seems as if the only place where we can agree is in our agreement as to how we should differ. So it is no surprise that establishing means through which differences can be expressed has commanded such attention. The idea of individual autonomy has become more and more important in a society which finds little else in which common cause can be made. A fresh focus on the concept of 'informed consent' as the bottom line of patients' rights seems a natural development. Is this not the key to a stable yet pluriform medical culture?

The only protection for the patient's conscience in a situation of contested ethical values lies in a right to oversee the ethical options available to the physician. Yet this – like the pressure for 'lay' involvement in ethical committees and the growing tendency to invoke judicial review of clinical judgments should be understood as a defensive response to the inevitable uncertainty produced by the absence of an ethical consensus at the heart of medical practice. Of course, in many situations the question is not simple. It is difficult to define the levels of 'freedom' and 'information' required for there to be informed consent. The Principle plainly depends on some notion of sufficiency: the patient's decision-making must be sufficiently free and also sufficiently informed; it can be absolutely neither, and there will be serious limits on the material with which the patient can be expected to be familiar in order to make an informed choice. We make this point since it raises a question-mark against the easy notion that there is a simple choice between autonomy for the patient and medical paternalism. For who but the physician can bear responsibility for informing the patient? And what level of information must there be? There are special situations which require special handling if the patient is incompetent or if giving the patient key information could be harmful.

The more fundamental question relates to the typical case and the fact that it is generally the physician who must himself give the patient whatever opportunity there may be to opt in or out of a treatment regime. The one who diagnoses and prescribes will also be the one who offers the patient the choice, and on whose briefing the patient's decision will crucially depend. But this raises the whole question of the doctor-patient relationship in post-Hippocratic medicine. We have argued that Hippocratism represented a revolutionary re-modeling of that relationship, on lines which placed the interests of the patient at the centre of the medical enterprise. The special difficulty raised by post-Hippocratic pluralism in medical values is that this philanthropic concept of medicine, with its inbuilt assumptions about where the patient's interests lie, is placed in jeopardy. With the retreat from the Hippocratic consensus there arises the potential for deep conflict between rival perceptions of where the patient's good is to be found. It puts the physician in the new situation of having to subordinate his own concept of the best interests of the patient to the patient's own.

We know that the antique culture out of which Hippocratism emerged was not a culture of consensus, least of all in medicine. Not only was

Hippocratism born in a pluralist culture, it was from the start controversial, its Oath the manifesto of a small minority intent on radical reform of contemporary medical practice.

So it cannot be said that Hippocratic practice depends on a consensus culture, however traumatic the breakdown of that consensus is proving.

This assumption is often made, by critic and defender alike. The minority and reformist character of ancient Hippocratism suggests something different. It first rose to prominence and, finally, to a position of unchallenged supremacy, as a radically controversial alternative to the accepted canons of medical practice in the ancient world. But this is not how we have come to perceive Hippocratic values, since we find ourselves at the end of a long tradition of consensus in our society. It is hardly surprising that our consensus experience has long been projected into pre-Christian Greece as the basis of the Hippocratic myth of late antique medicine. Yet if Hippocratism does not depend upon consensus within society, or indeed within the medical profession, on what does it depend? At its heart lies a more modest consensus, between doctor and patient. The Hippocratic idea of the doctor-patient relationship carries with it specific values to which they are both alike committed. Irrespective of consensus in society, this community of values between physician and patient is central to the Hippocratic tradition.

The character of these values ensured the rapid spread of Hippocratism in the ancient world, and its unchallenged dominance in the ensuing medical tradition of the West. For these values, while they have been called paternalistic (they are defined by the physician's own distinctive tradition and packaged together with his clinical skills), set the patient's interests above everything else. Its values found wide acceptance. We have seen that they can be, summed up as two: sanctity and philanthropy, and they are interlinked. By ruling out life-taking, and defining the task of the physician as that of the healer, the character of the physician's philanthropy is defined in the plainest terms. The Hippocratic Oath serves as the physician's calling-card: by defining the character of his medicine it also defines him, the professional, whose life and art are devoted to the care of his patients.

This leads us to an important distinction between Hippocratic medicine and 'paternalism' in general. Paternalism typically implies an assertion of authority, a claim (on the doctor's part) to the right to impose his decisions on the patient. Yet that is not Hippocratism. The Hippocratic physician claims no such right, except as he is himself subject to the philanthropic and professional demands of medicine. It is these demands which involve him in accepting a distinct ethical framework as the basis for his practice. This knitting together of technical skill and moral commitment defines Hippocratism and, in turn, the limits of the physician's freedom of action. Hippocratic 'paternalism' is nothing other than that limitation. So it is primarily the *physician* who is not free to take his own decisions. He is bound by Hippocratic philanthropy. The patient remains free to accept or reject his clinical judgment, but just as he may not demand treatment which the physician judges clinically inappropriate, so he may not require ethical conduct which the physician has forsworn. This covenantal welding of patient and physician involves no submission on the part of the patient to any subjective judgment of the physician. Hippocratism represents predictable medicine, medicine that is ethically candid. It is controversial today, and it was controversial when the Hippocratic manifesto first burst upon the ancient medical establishment in the second half of the fourth century BC. But it has always been candid.

In fact, the key to the Hippocratic idea of the relationship between doctor and patient lies in the notion of covenant. There is much current interest in such a model of the relationship yet, as we have seen, its roots lie in the Oath itself. Here the most distinctive feature is its three-dimensional character, which embraces the physician's covenant with his professional colleagues and his covenant with his patient, both alike rooted in his primary covenant with God. The covenantal model of the doctor-patient relationship is especially relevant at a time when pluralism and the assertion of patient autonomy threaten to reduce it to something wholly contractual. Of course there are contractual elements in this, as in every professional relationship, but they have never before threatened to become determinative of the relationship. It is a relationship between two persons, doctor and patient. The contractual analogy always threatens to distort what is fundamentally personal. The elements of remuneration and accountability, if taken as determining rather than subordinate factors, actually make the practice of medicine impossible.

It is in this light that we see the Hippocratic relationship emerging from the shadows of paternalism. A contractual reduction of medical care inevitably brings such a charge in its wake since, if the governing analogy is that of the commercial contract, there can be no place for any values which have not been negotiated. If, by contrast, it is understood that the Hippocratic covenant determines the pattern of the relationship, for doctor as for patient, the physician is no longer seen as paternal. Patient and physician come together into the Hippocratic enterprise.

So Hippocratic medicine can be charged with paternalism in only a special sense. The doctor is not himself making decisions for what he perceives to be the patient's good, on behalf of the patient. He has freely indentured himself into Hippocratic medicine. Yet his patients have also freely invited him into the therapeutic relationship. They are partners together in the Hippocratic covenant.

What of the future?

It may seem provocative to ask the question: *Is there a future for medicine?* At a time when advances in medical technique are announced with dulling frequency, if it is understood as an exercise in technique there can hardly be a doubt that the future of medicine is bright with extraordinary promise. While the high-tech medicine of the West stands in ever greater contrast to the struggles of primitive medical cultures in so much of the world, the continued upward progress of medical technique in contexts where the economy can support it offers the prospect of regular major breakthroughs in treatment. So is medicine's future not assured?

It all depends, of course, on what we mean by medicine. There are two questions, not one. First, is there a future for the Hippocratic tradition? We have sought to define 'medicine' in terms of Hippocratism. For all the medicine we have known is that marriage of technique and value which is the hallmark of the Hippocratic tradition. Moreover, the distinctly professional character of the medicine we know is, as we have seen, a Hippocratic legacy. If by medicine we mean the professional enterprise which holds a high place in society, it is Hippocratism of which we speak. The idea of professional medicine is known only in this single tradition. We have yet to see another medicine than that of Hippocrates.

Does it have a future? Its seamless dress is unraveling, technique is being divorced from values, and clinical skill imparted without regard to moral commitment. The leadership of the profession is increasingly in the hands of a generation which knew not Hippocrates. Yet this is not so of all of the profession, its individual practitioners and its institutions. We have noted the deep-seated conservatism of all human institutions, and the professions above all, a conservatism which has the double effect of both delaying fundamental change and once it is in progress of camouflaging its significance. Once such an institution begins to shift its position, a condition of the success of the shift is that it should not be acknowledged either to the public, or to members or even leaders of the profession itself. It may be left to a later generation to admit to what has happened and to recognize the new perspective as new. By that time, of course, it will already have taken on the appearance of a tradition.

Yet there will be those who do not shift. Their stand for what has suddenly become a minority position will not be easy. In maintaining what they consider to be the profession's proper values they discover that they are isolated. Those who are most strongly wedded to the tradition discover that the tradition has itself been marginalized, and them with it. Yet the new mainstream of the profession stands in an ambiguous position, since it cannot acknowledge that what is happening represents a shift at all. So not only will the minority experience a growing feeling of isolation, which may ultimately be profound, they will find their sense of identity called into question. And this process will be heightened by their gradual recognition that in their desire to conform they have fallen out of step with the very profession of which they have been loyal and conservative members. The ground has shifted from under them. As a result, they will be treated by their colleagues as disturbers of the professional peace. There is nothing so rigid in its conformities as a profession: it is this which makes it so resistant to change. Yet, when change comes, it outflanks the position of those who were so recently the staunchest defenders of the profession and its values. Once they were conservatives, conserving the professional tradition. They are suddenly cast as dissidents, whose role within the profession must be radical and, in principle, subversive. Whether they can continue to play any significant role within the community of the profession depends crucially on their level of awareness of what is going on. Their insight into their new situation is vital to their survival as an identifiable, if minority, group within the profession, and therefore to the continuance of the paradigm conflict which it represents. Of course, it is for this very reason that the profession itself will seek to undermine their influence, since the profession cannot admit how great a change is taking place. There is no option open to the profession but to re-cast the minority in an unflattering role.

The process is likely to go further. Though it will include some of the profession's leaders of a generation before, the minority may be stigmatized as unprofessional and its maintenance of what it claims to be the 'old values' regarded as incompatible with good standing in the profession today. It is likely to bring the profession into disrepute, since its charge that the profession has broken with essentials of its own tradition is deeply threatening to the status in society of the profession as a whole. The wheel has turned full circle. The defenders of Hippocratism are pushed to the margins of medicine, and regarded as a threat to its best interests.

Little by little, the profession is repudiating its Hippocratic origins, though doing so little conscious of the scope or significance of the (seemingly) piecemeal changes in policy. Of course, there are individuals within the profession, some of them highly placed, who know the meaning of these developments; and who have consistently promoted the new policies. But the candid public discussion of the values of the new medicine and the open repudiation of Hippocratism have not lain with the profession, but with those writers (mostly from outside the ranks of medicine itself) whose vision of the new medicine is clear, conscious and unashamed. Many within the profession are altogether unaware of their work, and others regard them as extreme: their proposals for fundamental ethical restructure-ing are generally discounted. The profession does not see (or admit) that what these prophets of the new medicine seek is already in train. Their vision of a medicine set free from Hippocratic trammels is beginning to be realized. So, though few physicians will counsel the killing of handicapped neonates or Alzheimer's patients, the new ethical writers can see that the seeds of such a policy have already been sown in the ambiguity which, above all, characterizes the medical approach to such situations. These writers are unafraid to propose in the place of such ambiguity a consistent and candid alternative to Hippocratic practice. The profession, as they can see, is quietly preparing to shift its ground, though with as little acknowledgment as possible of what is in progress; even to itself.

Of course, in breaking with its Hippocratic roots, the profession is merely following the values of the society which it serves. The relation between society's values and professional values can be complex. The conservative character of a profession will always tend to leave professional values behind those of the rest of society. There will be a time-lag between shifts in the values of society as a whole and the equivalent and ensuing shifts in the values of such institutions as the professions.

It is not that medicine has forced the pace of change. Rather, in its own special sphere, medicine is working through those fundamental shifts in value which have already begun to be widely accepted by society at large. Of course, there are other conservative institutions in society which are equally resistant to change. Societies do not change their perspectives tidily, and this has helped to obscure the significance of what is taking place in medicine. The fact that society has moved on, while medical values have (until recently) remained largely unchanged, is confusing to the observer, who gains the impression that the new general values have left professional values largely untouched. The final significance of the changes in general values, in this case for medicine, is hidden from view. At the same time, key members of the profession, as their own thinking is suffused by society's changed perspectives on a range of questions, are unsurprised to find professional values in flux. It seems a natural progress to bring them into harmony with the assumptions now widely held outside the profession. What is little recognized is that, in the process, professional values are not simply being adjusted but undergoing a revolution.

Indeed, we may discern a two-stage process which first delays, but finally has the effect of facilitating so fundamental a shift in values. First, despite shifts in society at large, the conservative character of the profession safeguards its internal values. Those who rely on the profession from outside are reassured that its values remain constant and seemingly unaffected; and that in turn may actually encourage the processes of change outside. Yet the old values are conserved by the profession for only a limited period. A new generation seeks to adjust the values of the profession to those round about; to catch up with what has been going on outside. The point of this analysis is to draw attention to the fact that at no point does the profession squarely face the issues posed by the move to a new set of values. Its conservative and enclosed character, far from protecting it, has the ironic effect of opening the profession wide to the new values. Only a minority of its members resist, since only a minority are out of step with the majority opinion in society, of which, of course, the members of the profession are made up. Their motivation must be strong. The most straightforward motive is that of religious convictions, which involve adhesion to a special set of values which may be expected to be at variance with those of society round about. Such an awareness of the likelihood of conflict between the values of the individual and those of society is a necessary ingredient in opening the eyes of a minority within the profession to the significance of fundamental change. It is that same awareness which will encourage the development of a self-consciously dissident tradition, even among the most conservative members of the profession.

What is the future of medicine? We pose the question differently now. If the future of Hippocratism is bleak, what future has post-Hippocratic medicine, the 'new medicine'? Clearly, in one sense, the future would seem to belong to post-Hippocratism-to the new identity in which the medicine is being clothed. But is this new medicine a viable, stable enterprise? Will its form be recognizable as that of a professional discipline, however unlike Hippocratism it may prove? Does the new medicine have a future, or will it come apart at the seams as value and technique, joined together by Hippocrates, are inexorably put asunder?

New for Old: The Story So Far The essence of Ludwig Edelstein's reconstruction of Hippocratic origins is the context he finds for the Oath in the Pythagoreanism of the later fourth century BC. Hippocratic medicine was then, and for some time later, the tradition of a small minority within the wider medical community. This overturned the assumption that Hippocratism was typical of the medical practice of ancient Greece, and casts Hippocratism in a new and vital contemporary role.

Edelstein spoke of the Oath as a 'manifesto'. Yet it was a manifesto for reform, and reform was sorely needed in the medicine of the day. These were controversial values when the Oath first demanded them, and their controversial character has now been, dramatically rediscovered.

The fusion of Hippocratic and Judaeo-Christian ethics ensured the final triumph of Hippocratism in the Graeco-Roman world and its establishment as the medical tradition of the West. We have seen in Nazi Germany the one major anti-Hippocratic intrusion into that western medical tradition, when Hippocratic values were disdained by a medical profession which embraced the involuntary euthanasia of the handicapped and thereby prepared the way, in technique as well as ethics, for the programme of 'involuntary euthanasia' which was the Holocaust. And then, with so large a number of human beings wholly at their disposal, without rights in law and with none to speak for them, the German medical-scientific establishment was associated in the human experimental programmes at Auschwitz and elsewhere.

Such anti-Hippocratism was overtly disavowed by the world medical community in the aftermath of war. The fruit of international reaction to the medical trials at Nuremberg was the Declaration of Geneva, which sought to re-instate Hippocratism and re-establish the historic values of the western medical tradition. Yet, in sad reality, the Declaration was something else. It marked not the re-birth of Hippocratism but the beginnings of a post-Hippocratic decline. The Hippocratic guise in which this new secular and malleable medical philosophy was dressed served to obscure the profound change which its adoption symbolized. In reaction to the depredations' of the German physicians, the world medical community did indeed wish to register its horror and affirm its commitment to the substance of the

Hippocratic values. But it did so in a form considered appropriate to the mid-twentieth century, denying any transcendent, theistic ground for its ethics and thereby turning covenant into mere code.

As such, it has proved open to amendment. So it is no surprise that, in place of the sanctity of life, it speaks of 'utmost respect for life', in which the relative character of 'respect' is ironically recognized by it qualification with 'utmost'. The door was now open for mainstream, and not simply rogue, medicine to leave the Hippocratic path. In breaking with the three-dimensional character of medical values which is the product of the transcendent grounding of the ethics of the Oath, post-Hippocratism crucially abandoned one central tenet of the tradition: Its limited but firm conviction of the dignity of human nature. The Pythagoreans and Judaeo-Christian doctrines had this in common, that human life mattered because it was given by God. Since we are accountable to him for our use of human life, our own and others', we may take neither (whether in feticide, suicide, senicide or some other homicide). The general supremacy accorded to the interests of the patient – the idea of Hippocratic philanthropy – stemmed from this same principle.

The subtle switch from vertical to merely horizontal ethics, symbolized in the new form in which the Declaration of Geneva cast the substance of Hippocratic values, marked the definitive distancing of post-war medicine from the transcendent Hippocratism of the western tradition.

In consequence, the door was formally opened to the development of something quite new: Medicine after Hippocrates, the new in place of the old.

These are two fundamentally divergent understandings of the nature of medicine. In one it is a service, offering healing or, if that is not possible, palliation to the sick.

In the other, it is a means of serving the interests of the powerful, whether in their own healing, or in their destruction, or in the healing or destruction of others. Plainly, the practical overlap between the two is substantial. That partly accounts for the failure of so many to grasp the significance of the changes in progress. Yet the change has been made, and with the passage of time the logic of the new medicine is set to eclipse the vestiges of the old order of humane Hippocratism.

Before Hippocrates: Back to the Future As we have seen, Edelstein's re-discovery of the Pythagorean origins of the Hippocratic tradition reveals it as a radical, reformist movement. Outraged by the character of the medicine of their day, the first Hippocrates set out to offer an alternative: philanthropic medicine based on the sanctity of life. We know that those practices outlawed in the Oath were current in Greek antiquity. And while some of them would have been widely recognized as abuses such as the exploitation of the clinical situation to obtain sexual favors others were simply normal practice. We know this is true of both abortion and suicide-euthanasia. They are forbidden in the Oath since they were common features of the medicine of antiquity, not abuses but practices widely seen to lie within the range of appropriate clinical options. That was the character of pre-Hippocratic medicine.

It is interesting to note the anthropologist Margaret Mead's characterization of the transition to Hippocratic medicine, as she takes us back to the paradigm shift which marked the revolution in medical values with which the story began: 'the Hippocratic Oath marked one of the turning points in the history of man'.

She writes: 'For the first time in our tradition there was a complete separation between killing and curing. Throughout the primitive world the doctor and the sorcerer tended to be the same person. He with the power to kill had power to cure, including specifically the undoing of his own killing activities. He who had power to cure would necessarily also be able to kill.' But within Greek Hippocratism 'the distinction was made clear. One profession, the followers of Asclepius, were to be dedicated completely to life under all circumstances, regardless of rank, age, or intellect the life of a slave, the life of the Emperor, the life of a foreign man, the life of a defective child.'

This telling testimony to the unique historical significance of Hippocratism, from someone with an unparalleled understanding of primitive peoples, is highly significant, not least because its author is aware of the implications of what she writes for contemporary concerns. Margaret Mead regards the Hippocratic tradition as 'a priceless possession which we cannot afford to tarnish; yet "society always is attempting to make the physician into a killer – to kill the defective child at birth, to leave the sleeping pills beside the bed of the cancer patient'. It is 'the duty of society to protect the physician from such requests."

So the new is but a recrudescence of the pre-Hippocratic old. The new medicine emerges as a re-statement of those values which the Hippocratic physicians consciously sought to displace with their reforming manifesto. The new medicine is the medicine of new paganism, seeking once more to turn the physician into someone who can kill as well as cure, who has power over the lives of his patients, to heal and to destroy. 'Society is always attempting to make the physician into a killer,' and in the rise of the new medicine it is succeeding. Killing has been restored to clinical practice and the clock put back to the days before Hippocrates.

The Hippocratic Challenge What is to be done?
The first requirement is for those who seek to maintain the tradition to develop a clear sense of identity and direction, just like the first Hippocratics. From its inception, ancient Hippocratism was marked from inside and out by a sense of being a 'profession within a profession', a dissident self-consciousness. That was why the Oath was sworn. In our day, in the aftermath of consensus Hippocratic medicine, this will not be easy. Yet that is how the first Hippocratics reformed the ancient medical culture. If modern, post-Hippocratic medicine is to be reformed, and the covenantal, philanthropic enterprise to survive and flourish again, that is a prerequisite. These must be the twin goals of Hippocratic medicine today: firstly, to maintain the tradition, to keep Hippocratic medical practice alive at all costs (and they may prove to be high); and secondly to work for the recovery of the Hippocratic medical culture. If this seems a tall order today, it can have seemed no taller in pre-Hippocratic Greece. If the spectacular success of Hippocratism in determining the course of western medicine owed much to the rise of Christianity, we find ourselves today in a world in which the tides of faith both ebb and flow. It is a world which continues to recognize its debt to the Christian tradition. Where the post-Christian society is most strongly emerging, as in much of western Europe, the challenges that much greater. Where more conservative societies are preserving and defending the faith and its values (whether in the Irish Republic or the conservative religious segments of the USA) the salt of Hippocratism is salty still. In the new and increasingly Christian nations of the Third World there is a ripe opportunity for the Hippocratic rooting of developing medical traditions.

Yet it is important to realize that this is not a narrowly religious question. Of course, as we have noted, those physicians who are most alarmed by the development of the new medicine and the collapse of the Hippocratic frontiers include many Christians, particularly Catholics and evangelicals. They will be at the forefront of the constant controversy which is entailed in the continuing paradigm debate keeping it open when it is in the interests of the new medicine that it should appear to be ended. Yet there are others who share the concern of Christians. Hippocratism is not

Christian medicine, however happily its central tenets have been married with Judaeo-Christian ethical concerns. Its first religious context, of course, was that of the Pythagorean paganism of late Greek antiquity. Christians, Jews and Muslims have readily adopted the religious–ethical structure of Hippocratism and meshed it into their own distinctive understandings of medicine.

The Hippocratic cause is broad, and that has been part of its genius – as is evidenced by its enormous influence in the Judaeo-Christian West and in mediaeval Arab medicine. At its root, as we have noted, lies a transcendent reference beyond the human medical situation in the theistic grounding of its ethics and the covenant commitment of the physician to his God. The physician is accountable and perceives the value of human life to derive from its Creator. Though that statement is modest, for the Christian, the Jew and the Muslim there is a wealth of theological content with which it may be filled. Yet its appeal is also to those whose religious commitment is less explicit, and to those who have none.

That is why Hippocratism could spread through various of the philosophical schools of Greece before ever it was borne to victory in western thought on the shoulders of the Church.

A vital point must not be missed here, for it would be easy for the theistic grounding of Hippocratic values to be taken to imply their irrelevance for those who deny any such religious commitment, though opinion poll evidence continues to suggest that only a small minority deny that they have any faith at all, even in a society as advanced in its secularization as that of the UK. Deny the theism, it is said, and what need have we of the ethics which sought in theism their justification? Only this: that the secular societies of the West have fallen heir to much of the ethical substance of their theistic tradition. That need not be an argument for theism, but it offers a powerful argument against the dismissal of those humane values which the tradition has bequeathed us.

This is underlined when the implications of some of the 'new ethics' are worked through and contrasted with the concern for the weak, the powerless, the sick, the young and the old which has marked the western tradition at its best and most consistent. As general social values, we shall not readily let go of these marks of the humane society; yet they are the values also of Hippocratism. It is in medical ethics that the dignity and rights of human beings have begun to be systematically threatened. The correlation of changing values in medicine with values which our post-Christian communities are eager to maintain in society at large offers a growing point in our understanding of the implications of the post-Hippocratic medical culture.

The way in which we have sought to address two of the key issues in this debate offers an example of the kind of argument between conflicting paradigms which is both legitimate and potentially effective. For what does any explanatory hypothesis claim? It claims to offer the best available explanation the evidence, the best available model for understanding reality the area under discussion.

If – as here – it is offered as a basis of professional practice, it must claim to offer the most coherent and effective understanding of things (specifically, in this case, of people) as they are. Hippocratic ethics have a theistic grounding, that they claim to be true - true to human nature, the most consistent coherent explanation of human nature as a basis for medical practice. Alternatives are not simply to be regarded as in error, they are to be subject to the most searching criticism to demonstrate why they fail to be equally consistent, equally coherent, why they fail to do justice to human nature and to medical practice.

That is the context in which we have discussed the question the nature of the embryo, probing the incoherence of Singer's radical alternative and seeking to show that, even on his own terms, his model of human nature, with its crucial dependence on 'morally relevant characteristics' was untenable; how it was in fact congruent with the very Nazi elitism its author sought to criticize. Again, in our discussion of euthanasia we drew attention to the incoherence of the central notion of voluntaryism which lies at the heart of any credible case for a humane euthanasia policy. In developing these critiques we have not been merely point-scoring, but rather putting post-Hippocratic models up for comparison with the tradition, setting in Kuhnian terms paradigm against paradigm, seeking to show the appeal of one perspective by denying that the other offers a coherent alternative understanding of reality. So also, in some other matters such as the coherence of patient autonomy as an alternative to what is widely seen as Hippocratic paternalism.

At no point have we offered an argument from faith (Pythagorean, Christian or other!); though Christians and Pythagoreans will have their own arguments for taking up these same positions. Much has been written about the implications for argument of the kind of sketching of competing hypotheses with which Kuhn's name is especially associated. It is certainly not intended to suggest that the relative circularity which this understanding recognizes implies a vicious circularity, since competing accounts are competing accounts of things as they are. It is in their rival attempts to portray and interpret things as they are that competing paradigms do battle for the allegiance of our understanding. Whatever the theistic context of the Pythagorean-Christian medical tradition, it has all along been offered and defended as a way of doing medicine in accord with human nature as it actually is; and in contrast to ways which do not accord with human nature as it actually is, and also (and accordingly) which will not work. For beyond any other human pursuit, medicine is the art of human nature, and any medical model, Pythagorean or Singerian, will be suffused with covert or candid assumptions about who we are and what are the boundaries of the 'we'. How could it be anything other?

The practical implications are clear. Christians and others who share the Hippocratic values are called to follow in the footsteps the first Hippocratic physicians, and to assume the dissident and reforming role which once was theirs. The wheel has nearly turned full circle. In the West the Christian centuries seem to be drawing to a close. Society is returning, slowly but substantially, to the values of the old paganism, and it is no surprise that the "new" medicine, in particular, is the reappearance in sophisticated garb of pre-Hippocratic pagan medical values.

In so far as this is a debate within medicine, the aim at every point must be to force those who occupy the emerging mainstream of the medical profession on to the defensive together with their ethical apologists. They must be asked to justify their post-Hippocratism, to be candid in their overthrow of centuries of human medical tradition, and they must be exposed as they seek by sleight of hand to claim professional and ethical precedent for their revolutionary programme.

Critics of the new medicine must gain a broad perspective on these developments. While it is necessary to concentrate on particular questions which focus the clash of these two medical cultures abortion and the killing of handicapped newborns for example it is vital that sight is not lost of the context of these flashpoints in the general development of the new medicine. Above all, we must re-assert the transcendent, covenantal character of Hippocratism as the only ground of humane, philanthropic medical practice. It was its simple attractiveness to doctor and patient alike, arising out of its patent appropriateness to human nature, that took the convictions of a 'small and isolated group' to a position of unrivalled dominance in twenty centuries of western medicine.

Perhaps it will again.

CHAPTER 7

TOWARD A MORE NATURAL MEDICINE

By

Patrick Guinan, MD

In 1985 Leon Kass published a book, "Toward a More Natural Science."[1] In it he defined natural as "true to life as found and lived."[2] He further discussed "teleology, Darwinism, and the place of man"[3] and concluded that nature has purpose and that the Hippocratic Oath repeatedly emphasized the fact that the physician must assist nature to maintain health, and in doing so the physician will be ethical. His discussions of medicine apply these principles to the relationship between the doctor and the patient.

The topic of what is "nature" and how its insights apply to human behavior, in this instance medicine, are particularly relevant. Although we live in, and benefit from, a modern scientific culture there has been an increasing unease with the dehumanizing aspects of seemingly out of control technology and the resultant mass materialistic consumerism. This

---

1   Kass Leon: Toward More Natural Science: Biology and Human Affairs. The Free Press, NY, 1985.
2   Ibid: p. xxi.
3   Ibid: pp.249-278.

unease is reflected in a growing concern with environmental issues and, in medicine, with the rapid growth in alternative or non-traditional medicine. Dr. Kass's reflections on "natural science" are particularly relevant.

Kass observes that nature, far from being simply the result of evolution and blind chance, as modern positivistic science has taught our culture, tells us that our concerns for justice, freedom, and knowledge itself, indicate that human beings have a self evident non-material dimension. This human aspect of nature includes ethics and, in medicine, is perhaps best the Hippocratic medical ethical tradition.

While we are most familiar with the Greek medical tradition as reflected in today's Western bioethical guidelines, there are several other major cultural traditions: Moslem, Hindu, Chinese and others. These traditions developed from human experience; the experience of sickness, suffering, and death being one of the most primal and universal. In all societies certain members, physicians, were designated as proficient in healing and a basic doctor-patient relationship was recognized. While initially there were religious and magic overtones, in all major cultures the physician appears to have observed nature and developed objective clinical criteria to diagnose and treat human disease. In dealing with illness the physician and patient have historically worked in conformity with nature.

The purpose of this paper is to 1) Describe Kass's understanding of a "natural" science. 2) Explain the relationship between nature and the medical ethic, and finally 3) Explore the transcultural conformity to this ethic.

I. A natural science For Kass, who in addition to being a physician, is also a scientist (having a doctorate in biochemistry), nature is marvelous in its many manifestations of purposiveness. Throughout the animal kingdom there are innumerable examples of the integration of form and function to achieve an end benefiting the involved species. There is a harmony between the environment and the accommodations of various life forms, up to and including the human. Nature and mankind have coexisted harmoniously until quite recently when our technology appears to have caused environmental damage.

Unfortunately the Enlightenment challenged and changed the symbiotic relationship between man and nature with a new understanding of science. Kass observes that modern science measures the singular and the material and does not observe the bigger picture, the tendency of nature toward purpose and fulfillment. He notes that the tension between the cult of modern science and the understanding of practically all prior human cultures began about three hundred years ago when Roger Bacon and Rene Descartes projected "the vision of the mastery of nature."[4] For all of recorded history prior to the Enlightenment man accommodated to, and conformed with, nature. With the scientific discoveries in chemistry, physics and biology it appeared that man need no longer be subservient to, but could now control and dominate nature. The scientific understanding of physiology, pathology, and particularly pharmacology seemed to confirm this mastery of man over nature in the field of medicine as well. This development, coincidentally, has profound cultural implications with a decline in the influence of transcendent religions and a rise in the spirit of human autonomy.

But can nature be mastered? The modern age, or era of the Enlightenment, appears to be in decline and we are now entering a postmodern time. Our attempt to master nature has resulted in environmental problems perhaps the most serious of which are atmospheric imbalances resulting in apparent global warming. It appears that we must be more in conformity with nature rather than dominating it.

Kass counters the Enlightenment science of blind chance with a more "natural science," or as he defines it, a science "true to life as found and lived." This world can be science that looks beyond atoms, molecules and genes and sees purpose and teleology. We look at human history and experience, and note rationality and freedom, but also a sense of right and wrong, which is synonymous with morality and ethics.

In summary, Dr. Kass tells us that if we reflect on our experience we realize that nature has purpose, is intelligible, and our actions have moral consequences.

For Kass the harmonious interface between nature and man is nowhere better exemplified than in medicine. The physician works with nature to the benefit of the patient.

II. Nature and medical ethics Kass's plea for a more natural science or a science "true to life as found and lived" as opposed to a science intent on control or a "mastery of nature" receives impetus from his understanding of medicine. The goal of medicine is promoting the health of the patient. By

---

4   Ibid: p. 2.

health Kass means "the well working of the organism as a whole."[5] While the newer developments in pharmacology and science are valuable they should be compatible with the natural human condition which conforms with "a natural science." Medicine must be "true to life as found and lived." Human beings are more than physical components; they are persons. Greek medicine realized this and incorporated the more natural science into the Hippocratic Oath.

The Oath assumes that medicine is a practical art and that it is a moral art. It is an art because in treating a sick patient the physician diagnoses and treats by the active observation of symptoms and discovery of signs, and then intervenes with dietetics or pharmacology. Medicine is a moral art because the Oath is specific as to what a physician can, and most importantly cannot, do: in other words what is ethical. A physician first and foremost cannot harm (primum non nocere). But there are many other proscriptions. Among others, the physician also cannot break a confidence, nor can he/she take sexual advantage of a patient. Interestingly, Hippocratic morality negates social status: a physician must treat a slave as he would a freeman. Medicine is preeminently a moral art.

Kass notes that the wisdom of the Hippocratic Oath resides in the fact that it directs the physician to assist living nature. "The physician is an assistant to nature"[6] and more importantly "the doctor is nature's cooperative ally and not its master." A doctor's relationship with his patient is a moral or ethical relationship. Medicine is a moral art. Kass feels so strongly that medicine embodies the ideal of the "natural" in its ethical principles, as enumerated in the Oath, that he states that the "ethic of medicine rightly understood, could come to be the basis of ethics generally."[7]

Although the Hippocratic Code guided physicians for 2500 years, for a variety of reasons, the imperatives it once carried has been diminished. This is unfortunate because the Hippocratic Oath has insights that can benefit both physicians and patients today.

Summarizing, Dr. Kass believes that the Hippocratic Oath is a watershed ethical document. It contains several moral imperatives derived from insights into human nature: among others are included: respect persons, treat others equally and finally do not harm. Medicine is a moral art and the Hippocratic imperatives are the basis of much of human ethics.

---

5   Ibid: p. 174.
6   Ibid: p. 233.
7   Ibid: p. 239.

That the ethics of the healing art are reflected in nature as "found and lived" is demonstrated by the consistency of medical ethical codes across cultural boundaries.

III. Transcultural Affirmation There are many similarities of the various medical ethical codes of the major human cultures.[8] In general, the medical ethical traditions of all major cultures have tended to respect nature. They have attempted to find balance and accommodate to natural forces. This may have been, in part, because they couldn't effectively influence nature, and therefore had no choice. Be that as it may, these cultures saw life as good and to be respected. In general, abortion, suicide, and euthanasia were forbidden. Man was expected to live in harmony with nature.

While nature tends toward wholeness, disease, whether spontaneous or self inflicted has been the lot of humankind from before recorded history. Initially men attributed physical disease to divine intervention. In primitive societies the medicine man or shaman was a combined physician and priest but as cultures developed a clear distinction was made between the two. Early recorded history in both Mesopotamia and Egypt[9] indicates that physicians were clearly distinguished from priests. Indeed before there were oaths to be sworn to by doctors there were laws, such as those of Hammurabi and Imhotep, governing the physician's conduct.

It is possible to compare Greek, Christian, Jewish, Moslem, Hindu and Chinese traditions according to the four principles elucidated in the eight paragraphs of the Hippocratic Oath. These are 1. the invocation of a higher power, 2. the resolve not to harm the patient, 3. respect for the privacy and confidentiality of the patient and finally, 4. regard for the profession and one's teacher.

The Greek medical tradition, associated with Hippocrates (460-377 BC) and elaborated by his followers originated in the golden age of Greek intellectual genius. The fact that the Hippocratic corpus may have been influenced by Pythagorean philosophy is somewhat immaterial because it was the former ethical tradition which was eventually associated with Greek medicine which has had a profound influence on subsequent Christian, Jewish and Moslem physicians.

8   Etziony H: The Physician's Creed. Charles Thomas Publishers, Springfield, IL, 1973.
9   Amundson D and Ferngren G: Near and Middle East. In Encyclopedia of Bioethics, Reich WT, Editor, Simon and Schuster Macmillan, New York, pp. 1440-1445, 1995.

Roman medicine, while technically advanced by Galen and others, retained the Hippocratic ethic which in turn was adopted by the Christian and subsequent European physicians after Constantine's Edict in 313 AD. St. Jerome commented favorably on the Hippocratic Oath.[10] Jewish medicine, while conforming to biblical strictures, was clinical in nature and not religious. Maimomides' prayer incorporated the four Hippocratic principles.[11] Moslem medicine was strongly influenced by the Greek schools of the eastern Mediterranean. The most recent formulation of the Islam Code of Medical Ethics is essentially a paraphrase of the Hippocratic Oath.[12] It can appropriately be said that the Christian (or European), Jewish and Moslem medical communities continued, practically intact, the Hippocratic ethic.

The Hindu physician's code[13] begins with an acknowledgment of the sacred fire and admonishes the physician not to injure or desert the patient even at the risk of his (the physician's) own livelihood or even life. It describes at length the doctors obligation to the patient and his family, and also to his teachers and medical colleagues.

The Chinese physicians' code[14] begins by recognizing the need for divine guidance. It continues by urging the physician to consider the patient's misery his own, and to relieve the patient's distress disregarding any inconvenience to himself. The physician should be competent and care for all patients, rich and poor.

It will be noted that medical codes of the various cultures tend to follow the outline of the Hippocratic Oath. There is a respect for nature and a tendency to work with nature to the betterment of the patient. The ethic of the codes is based on an acknowledgment of a divine authority and is mediated by virtue based on upright personal conduct. The physician becomes special by diligent learning, exemplary behavior, a respect for life and nature, and a recognition of the sacred.

Kass's observation about the Hippocratic Oath can be extrapolated as well to the medical codes of other great cultures. Medical ethics, as distilled through the wisdom of the great cultures and religions, reflects the natural tendency to respect life and do no harm. The interaction of

10   Amundson D.W: Early Christianity. Ibid. pp. 1516-1522, 1995.

11   Friedwald H: The Jews and Medicine. Johns Hopkins Press, Baltimore, 1944.

12   Hathout H: Contemporary Arab World. In Encyclopedia of Bioethics, Reich WT, Editor, Simon and Schuster Macmillan, New York, pp. 1452-1457. 1995.

13   Memon H and Haberman HF: A Medical Students Oath of Ancient India, Med Hist. 14:295-299, 1970.

14   T'ao Lee: Medical Ethics in Ancient China. Bull Hist Med 13:268, 1943.

a knowledgeable empathetic physician and a suffering patient represent one of the oldest, most profound, and ongoing of human experiences. It behooves physicians and future physicians to reflect on and absorb Kass's insights into a more natural medicine. As Dr. Kass observed, this medical ethic could be a paradigm for ethics in general.

CHAPTER 8

HIPPOCRATES SEDUCED

By

Patrick C. Beeman

In solemnly reciting the short Hippocratic Oath upon his graduation from medical school (it is about 340 to 380 words long, depending on the translation), the new physician declares, "I will follow that system of regimen which according to my ability and judgment, I consider for the benefit of my patients, and abstain from whatever is deleterious and mischievous."

Lest there be confusion about what constitutes mischief, the oath continues, "I will give no deadly medicine to anyone if asked, nor suggest any such counsel; and in like manor I will not give to a woman a pessary to produce abortion." These two foundational principles—prohibiting abortion and euthanasia--form the distinctive character of the oath.

You might imagine that when medical school graduates don their long white coats for the first time (medical students wear short ones), they all swear by "Apollo the physician, and Aesculapius" (some versions substitute "The All Mighty") to uphold these principles. After all, the American

Medical Association says that the Hippocratic Oath "has remained in Western Civilization as an expression of ideal conduct for the physician.

AMENDED HIPPOCRATES You would be wrong. Few medical schools require students to swear this oath upon graduation, opting instead for the recitation of a different, more politically palatable but less venerable pledge.

First administered in 1508 at the University of Wittenburg's medical school, the Hippocratic Oath gradually became incorporated as a formal graduation exercise on both sides of the Atlantic. In 1928, only 24 percent of schools in the United States and Canada administered the oath to their graduates, but after World War II, with the revelation of the atrocities committed by the Third Reich in the name of medical science, many more schools included an oath as part of the graduation rite.

In 1993, one hundred percent of American medical schools administered some oath to their graduates. However, few today actually use what could be called a "Hippocratic Oath," one that preserves its original intent while updating the language. Only 14 percent of the new oaths (Hippocratic or otherwise) prohibit euthanasia, only 8 percent proscribe abortion, and only 11 percent invoke God.

At my medical school, first-year students learn about a number of alternatives to the original Hippocratic Oath: Oath of Maimomides and the Prayer of Maimomides (neither by Maimomides); the Declaration of Geneva; and a handful of revisions of the Hippocratic Oath.

Both the Oath and the Prayer of Maimomides present life as something given by God to be served by the physician, stating, "Thou hast appointed me to watch over the life and death of Thy creatures." However, neither offers practical advice on how to live this out, and neither mentions abortion or euthanasia.

The Declaration of Geneva, formulated in 1949 by the World Medical Association, conscious of the Nuremburg trials, begins with a "solemn pledge" to consecrate one's life to the service of humanity. It then calls for such things as practicing medicine "with conscience and dignity" and maintaining patient confidentiality.

Importantly, it affirms, "I will maintain the utmost respect for human life from its beginning, even under threat, and I will not use my medical knowledge contrary to the laws of humanity. But it does not say, as does the Hippocratic Oath, "I will give no deadly medicine" nor "a pessary to produce abortion," and by formulating its practice in terms of an abstract "respect" and "the laws of humanity," it makes possible an approval of abortion or euthanasia.

Then there are the un-Hippocratic, modern revisions of the original oath, which reject, by absence or evasion, the traditional proscriptions on abortion and euthanasia. For instance, the British Medical Association's version — which is, as C. S. Lewis might have put it, an oath without a chest-proclaims "the special value of human life," yet immediately adds, "but I also know that the prolongation of human life is not the only aim of healthcare. Where abortion is permitted, I agree that it should take place only within an ethical and legal framework."

Another revision preserves the structure and some ideas of the original, though with the literary merit of a phonebook. It includes what looks like a euthanasia clause, declaring, "I swear to wield my art in such ways, and only in such ways, as serve to preserve sentient life in its myriad forms, or to allow such life to depart in dignity."

Still others, like Cornell Medical College's revision, simply leave out abortion and euthanasia.

DISCONNECTED DOCTORS I wonder whether the schools, and the students comfortable with the alternatives, consciously choose to ignore Hippocratic principles or whether their ignorance is just symptomatic of a greater cultural change since the time when the declarations of the oath were considered self-evident. Many of my colleagues seem to have whole-heartedly accepted the principles of the culture of death placed within our curriculum. The strident activism of our school's Medical Students for Choice is only a particularly sad example.

There is a disconnection between the traditional, Hippocratic idea of the medical profession serving life and the good, and an opposing, novel notion of the profession slowly being introduced into the medical curriculum. The alternative to the Hippocratic understanding of medicine is for medicine to become a tool for what some are calling the "new eugenics."

What sets medicine apart from pure science is that it asks the question, "What is the good for man?" rather than simply, "What is man?" Medicine can never he morally neutral, for the good of man is an inherently moral idea.

This is what makes the widespread acceptance by the profession - from the nadir of the first-year lecture hall to the heights of healthcare policymaking-of the morning-after pill, abortion, in vitro fertilization, contraception, euthanasia, and prenatal "screening" so horrifically disturbing. Such things cheapen human life where they do not destroy it outright.

During the lecture on medical oaths, one student asked in regard to the Hippocratic proscriptions on killing, "Wouldn't these preclude a doctor from prescribing the morning-after pill or advocating for euthanasia? The professor responded, "It would seem that way, wouldn't it?" Indeed it would.

Too many students—many without realizing it— are moved by lectures that covertly plant into their minds anti-life ideas. During our first course in medical school, we learned that physicians ought to feel compassion not because certain people were born with genetic diseases or birth defects such as Down syndrome or anencephaly, but because these individuals were not "screened" early enough (i.e., aborted).

Rather than presenting these lives as at least potentially good, the lecturers presented them as most definitely bad, as if this were self evident and the view that doctors naturally took. But the solution offered - aborting fetuses with known genetic defects—seems rather like the solution described by Chesterton as attempt-ing to "solve the problem of too few hats by lopping off heads."

Soon thereafter, we learned of the glories of diagnosing Down syndrome by ultrasound (more cost-effective than other prenatal rests), which could produce a nearly certain diagnosis. In this manner, a woman could very early be sped along the road to abortion, even though her child might nor really suffer from Down syndrome (not that killing him would be justified even if he were). The presumption seemed to be that children should, so far as is possible, be made to order.

THE TWO LOVES Nevertheless, many students do not think doctors should labor to destroy those they have promised to serve, when, they can devote themselves to comforting them and possibly, if only eventually, healing them. And as my limited experience—both as an applicant and as a student member of the admissions committee--has shown me, there are traditional elements in medical education that have perdured, such as medical students' reasons for wishing to become doctors.

As clichéd as it may sound, the answer applicants and students give to the question "Why medicine?" is invariably that they want to help people. I am convinced that most of my fellow students view the existence of disease as a moral imperative to take their intellectual talents and other abilities aid place them at the service of the most vulnerable among us.

Admittedly, a few students are in medicine exclusively in the hope of getting rich, satisfying intellectual curiosity, or gaining prestige. Still, when a student admits this, most of my friends groan or stare in disbelief at such an instrumental view of our profession, and remark that it would have been much easier for him to go into investment banking to get rich or the law to satisfy his intellectual curiosity.

But there is much in our medical schools and in our culture that suggests even to the idealistic that they may define their calling in different ways than did Hippocrates—by using their knowledge to screen out the "defective," for example. Thus, our medical schools offer their students bland, uncontroversial, inoffensive alternatives to the Hippocratic Oath and the ethics it embodies.

Elsewhere in the Hippocratic corpus we learn, "Where there is love of mankind, there is also love of the Art of medicine." Although this is nor always the case, where there is the art of medicine, with its inherent obligation to heal, there ought to be love of mankind, especially the poor, the sick, the aged, the unborn, and the handicapped.